Diagnosis and Management of Oral Mucosal Lesions

Editors

INDRANEEL BHATTACHARYYA
DONALD M. COHEN

ORAL AND MAXILLOFACIAL SURGERY CLINICS OF NORTH AMERICA

www.oralmaxsurgery.theclinics.com

Consulting Editor
RUI P. FERNANDES

May 2023 • Volume 35 • Number 2

ELSEVIER

1600 John F. Kennedy Boulevard • Suite 1800 • Philadelphia, Pennsylvania, 19103-2899

http://www.oralmaxsurgery.theclinics.com

ORAL AND MAXILLOFACIAL SURGERY CLINICS OF NORTH AMERICA Volume 35, Number 2
May 2023 ISSN 1042-3699, ISBN-13: 978-0-323-93925-6

Editor: John Vassallo; j.vassallo@elsevier.com
Developmental Editor: Jessica Nicole B. Cañaberal

Oral and Maxillofacial Surgery Clinics of North America (ISSN 1042-3699) is published quarterly by Elsevier Inc., 360 Park Avenue South, New York, NY 10010-1710. Months of issue are February, May, August, and November. Business and Editorial Offices: 1600 John F. Kennedy Blvd., Suite 1800, Philadelphia, PA 19103-2899. Periodicals postage paid at New York, NY and additional mailing offices. Subscription prices are $409.00 per year for US individuals, $785.00 per year for US institutions, $100.00 per year for US students/residents, $483.00 per year for Canadian individuals, $941.00 per year for Canadian institutions, $100.00 per year for Canadian students/residents, $535.00 per year for international individuals, $941.00 per year for international institutions and $235.00 per year for international students/residents. To receive student/resident rate, orders must be accompanied by name or affiliated institution, date of term, and the *signature* of program/residency coordinator on institution letterhead. Orders will be billed at individual rate until proof of status is received. Foreign air speed delivery is included in all *Clinics* subscription prices. All prices are subject to change without notice. **POSTMASTER:** Send address changes to *Oral and Maxillofacial Surgery Clinics of North America,* Elsevier Periodicals **Customer Service, 11830 Westline Industrial Drive, St. Louis, MO 63146. Tel: 1-800-654-2452 (U.S. and Canada); 314-447-8871 (outside U.S. and Canada). Fax: 314-447-8029.** E-mail: journalscustomerservice-usa@elsevier.com (for print support); journalsonlinesupport-usa@elsevier.com (for online support).

Reprints. For copies of 100 or more, of articles in this publication, please contact the Commercial Reprints Department, Elsevier Inc., 360 Park Avenue South, New York, NY 10010-1710. Tel.: 212-633-3874; Fax: 212-633-3820; Email: reprints@elsevier.com.

Oral and Maxillofacial Surgery Clinics of North America is covered in *MEDLINE/PubMed* (*Index Medicus*), *Science Citation Index Expanded (SciSearch®), Journal Citation Reports/Science Edition*, and *Current Contents®/Clinical Medicine.*

Contributors

CONSULTING EDITOR

RUI P. FERNANDES, MD, DMD, FACS, FRCS(Ed)
Clinical Professor and Chief, Division of Head and Neck Surgery, Program Director, Head and Neck Oncologic Surgery and Microvascular Reconstruction Fellowship, Departments of Oral and Maxillofacial Surgery, Neurosurgery, and Orthopaedic Surgery and Rehabilitation, University of Florida Health Science Center, University of Florida College of Medicine, Jacksonville, Florida, USA

EDITORS

INDRANEEL BHATTACHARYYA, DDS, MSD
Professor, Division and Laboratory Director, Oral and Maxillofacial Pathology, University of Florida College of Dentistry, Gainesville, Florida, USA

DONALD M. COHEN, DMD, MS, MBA
Professor Emeritus and Former Chair, Department of Oral and Maxillofacial Diagnostic Sciences, University of Florida College of Dentistry, Gainesville, Florida, USA

AUTHORS

SARAH AGUIRRE, DDS, MS
Assistant Professor of Oral and Maxillofacial Pathology, Department of Diagnostic Sciences, The University of Tennessee Health Science Center, College of Dentistry, Tennessee, USA

SAJA A. ALRAMADHAN, BDS
Assistant Professor, Department of Oral and Maxillofacial Diagnostic Sciences, University of Florida College of Dentistry, Gainesville, Florida, USA

LETICIA FERREIRA CABIDO, DDS, MS
Associate Professor, Department of Diagnosis and Oral Health, Diplomate, American Board of Oral and Maxillofacial Pathology, University of Louisville School of Dentistry, Louisville, Kentucky, USA

ASHLEY CLARK, DDS
University of Kentucky College of Dentistry, Lexington, Kentucky, USA

SARAH G. FITZPATRICK, DDS
Department of Oral and Maxillofacial Diagnostic Sciences, University of Florida College of Dentistry, Gainesville, Florida, USA

MARIA GEORGAKI, DDS, MSc, PhD
Elected Assistant Professor, Department of Oral Medicine and Pathology and Hospital Dentistry, School of Dentistry, National and Kapodistrian University of Athens, Greece

NADIM M. ISLAM, DDS, BDS
Professor and Residency Program Director, Department of Oral and Maxillofacial Diagnostic Sciences, University of Florida College of Dentistry, Gainesville, Florida, USA

JENNIE ISON, DMD
University of Kentucky College of Dentistry, Lexington, Kentucky, USA

IOANNIS KOUTLAS, DDS, MS
Associate Professor, Division of Oral and Maxillofacial Pathology, University of Minnesota School of Dentistry, Minneapolis, Minnesota, USA

MARK MINTLINE, DDS
WesternU Health Oral Pathology, Pomona, California, USA

VIMI SUNIL MUTALIK, BDS, MDS, MS, FRCD(C)
Assistant Professor, Department of Dental Diagnostic and Surgical Sciences, University of Manitoba Dr. Gerald Niznick College of Dentistry, Winnipeg, Manitoba, Canada

NIKOLAOS G. NIKITAKIS, MD, DDS, PhD
Professor, Head, Department of Oral Medicine and Pathology and Hospital Dentistry, School of Dentistry, National and Kapodistrian University of Athens, Greece

SCOTT M. PETERS, DDS
Assistant Professor, Division of Oral and Maxillofacial Pathology, Columbia University Irving Medical Center, New York, New York, USA

ELIZABETH M. PHILIPONE, DMD
Associate Professor, Division of Oral and Maxillofacial Pathology, Columbia University Irving Medical Center, New York, New York, USA

MÁRIO JOSÉ ROMAÑACH, DDS, MSc, PhD
Department of Oral Diagnosis and Pathology, School of Dentistry, Universidade Federal do Rio de Janeiro (UFRJ), Brazil

SHOKOUFEH SHAHRABI-FARAHANI, DDS, MS, DMSc
Associate Professor of Oral and Maxillofacial Pathology, Department of Diagnostic Sciences, The University of Tennessee Health Science Center, College of Dentistry, Memphis, Tennessee, USA

MOLLY HOUSLEY SMITH, DMD
Pathology and Cytology Laboratory, Lexington, Kentucky, USA

JASBIR D. UPADHYAYA, BDS, MSc, PhD
Assistant Professor, Department of Applied Dental Medicine, Southern Illinois University School of Dental Medicine, Alton, Illinois, USA

JAMIE WHITE, DMD
Assistant Professor, Oral and Maxillofacial Pathology, Department of Oral Maxillofacial Surgery and Pathology, University of Mississippi Medical Center, School of Dentistry, Jackson, Mississippi, USA

TINA R. WOODS, DMD
Associate Professor, Oral and Maxillofacial Pathology, Department of Stomatology, James B. Edwards College of Dental Medicine, Charleston, South Carolina, USA

RANIA H. YOUNIS, BDS, MDS, PhD
Clinical Associate Professor, Department of Oncology and Diagnostic Sciences, School of Dentistry, University of Maryland, Baltimore, Maryland, USA

Contents

Pigmented lesions are a common finding in the oral cavity. Oral pigmented lesions may range from solitary to multiple, pinpoint to diffuse, and have a variety of clinical implications. Nearly all solitary pigmented lesions require a biopsy to rule out mucosal melanoma. Oral mucosal melanoma has a grim prognosis and early discovery is of utmost importance. Multiple pigmented lesions in the oral cavity may indicate a systemic condition about which the patient may not be aware. The presentation and management of these various lesions is the focus of this article.

Nonodontogenic bacterial infections of the oral cavity are not a common finding in the United States. Nevertheless, there has been an increase in prevalence of certain bacterial sexually transmitted diseases, such as syphilis and gonorrhea, and conditions such as tuberculosis still pose a serious threat to certain segments of the population. Finally, given the uncommon nature and pathophysiology of these diseases, diagnosis is often delayed, resulting in more clinically significant disease and potential contamination of individuals. Thus, it is prudent that clinicians be familiar with these uncommon but potentially serious infectious diseases, so treatment can be instituted promptly.

The human herpesvirus (HHV) family is a group of enveloped DNA viruses containing 8 members known to produce oral mucosal lesions. Following initial exposure, which may result in symptomatic primary infection, the viruses establish latency within specific cells/tissues. After reactivation, herpesviruses can cause localized symptomatic or asymptomatic recurrent (secondary) infections or diseases. HHV may have a significant role in the cause of oral mucosal infectious diseases in immunocompromised patients. This article discusses the role of those herpesviruses that can induce oral mucosal lesions, with focus on the clinical features and treatment/management.

Lichenoid lesions involving the oral cavity present with an array of complex clinical manifestations and etiologies. The etiology ranges from local factors, systemic entities, and even autoimmune conditions. Several different types of lichenoid lesions may affect the oral cavity, and it is imperative that these are correctly diagnosed to ensure effective patient care. Lichenoid lesions such as chronic ulcerative stomatitis prove to be challenging as these are recalcitrant, present with overlapping features, require unique treatment and patients suffer a long time if not promptly diagnosed.

Plasma cell gingivitis (PCG) is an inflammatory condition that affects the gingival mucosa of the oral cavity. It is characterized by polyclonal dense plasma cell infiltrate in the connective tissue. Lesions do not respond to prophylactic treatment. Etiology is most likely hypersensitivity to certain antigens (eg, toothpastes, oral rinses, chewing gums, spices). Differential diagnosis of PCG includes reactive, granulomatous, and neoplastic lesions. The diagnostic workup is based on patient's history and the clinicopathologic correlation to rule out mimics of PCG. Dermatologic patch test may be indicated in chronic conditions to identify the allergen.

Oral fungal infections are opportunistic and due to impaired host resistance. The increasing number of immunosuppressed individuals contributes to rising numbers of mycoses worldwide, and the ease of global migration has allowed the geographic range of endemic mycoses to expand. Deep fungal infections can clinically mimic other pathologic conditions including malignancy. This review highlights the pathogenesis, clinical features, diagnosis, and treatment recommendations of eight fungal infections that can be encountered in the dental setting.

ORAL AND MAXILLOFACIAL SURGERY CLINICS OF NORTH AMERICA

SERIES OF RELATED INTEREST

Atlas of the Oral and Maxillofacial Surgery Clinics
www.oralmaxsurgeryatlas.theclinics.com

Dental Clinics
www.dental.theclinics.com

THE CLINICS ARE NOW AVAILABLE ONLINE!
Access your subscription at:
www.theclinics.com

Preface
Overview of Diagnosis and Management of Oral Mucosal Lesions

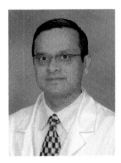   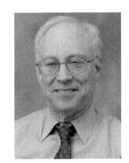

Indraneel Bhattacharyya, DDS, MSD   Donald M. Cohen, DMD, MS, MBA

Editors

Oral mucosal lesions not only are common but often present challenges in diagnosis, as many lesions have similar clinical features and require a detailed workup to find the cause. Furthermore, innocuous-appearing lesions may prove to be premalignant or malignant, not respond to classical treatment, and/or may represent oral manifestations of systemic disease. To diagnose a mucosal lesion, it is imperative that the clinician have a comprehensive list of possible entities in their differential diagnosis. Often clinicians fail to consider a wide range of possible entities, which could lead to a potential incorrect diagnosis or delayed treatment. The purpose of this issue is to enhance the diagnostic abilities of the practicing oral surgeon regarding various oral mucosal lesions and augment their management armamentariums. We hope to accomplish this by reviewing a host of common oral mucosal lesions from a wide variety of causes, including bacterial, viral, and mycotic to autoimmune ulcerative, lichenoid and lichen planus, and reactive and nonreactive lesions. Moreover, we introduce the reader to some newly described entities, such as chronic ulcerative stomatitis. Oral manifestations of systemic diseases, vesiculobullous diseases, and pigmented lesions are also discussed. Emphasis has been placed on information relevant to a practicing oral surgeon with a focus on new important entities, clinical pearls for diagnosis, and effective and newer treatments. In addition, multiple high-quality illustrations are included to highlight salient clinical presentations, which will aid in improving diagnostic skills. We also review critical clinical concepts, which are relevant to the entities discussed. We would like to thank the eighteen well-regarded and actively practicing oral pathologists from all over the United States for contributing to this eleven-article comprehensive review of oral and maxillofacial mucosal lesions. We, the editors, would also like to thank our colleagues, family members, and staff for their understanding and for allowing us to devote a significant amount of time to editing these articles.

Indraneel Bhattacharyya, DDS, MSD
Oral & Maxillofacial Pathology
University of Florida College of Dentistry
1395 Center Drive
Gainesville, FL 32610-0414, USA

Donald M. Cohen, DMD, MS, MBA
Department of Oral &
Maxillofacial Diagnostic Sciences
University of Florida College of Dentistry
1395 Center Drive
Gainesville, FL 32610-0414, USA

E-mail addresses:
ibhattacharyya@dental.ufl.edu (I. Bhattacharyya)
dcohen@dental.ufl.edu (D.M. Cohen)

Oral Maxillofacial Surg Clin N Am 35 (2023) ix
https://doi.org/10.1016/j.coms.2022.10.011
1042-3699/23/© 2022 Published by Elsevier Inc.

Pigmented Lesions of the Oral Cavity

Jennie Ison, DMD, Ashley Clark, DDS*

KEYWORDS

- Pigment • Melanoma • Melanotic • Nevus • Melanosis

KEY POINTS

- Pigmented lesions of the oral cavity are commonly encountered.
- Diffuse pigmented lesions of the oral cavity may be reactive or syndromic in nature.
- Isolated pigmented lesions of the oral cavity often require a biopsy to rule out melanoma.
- Rapidly expanding or changing characteristics of pigmented lesions necessitates a biopsy.

Pigmented lesions have various presentations in the oral cavity. Lesions may range from solitary to multiple, pinpoint to diffuse, and may have numerous different clinical implications. Nearly all solitary pigmented lesions require a biopsy to rule out oral mucosal melanoma; multiple lesions typically indicate a systemic condition. In this article, we will discuss the various common presentations of pigmented lesions of the oral cavity and their management.

ORAL MELANOTIC MACULE

The most common pigmented lesion of the oral cavity is the melanotic macule. Although any mucosal surface may be affected, the lower lip is the most common site. The buccal mucosa, palate, and gingivae are also frequently affected.[1–3] Although the cause is not known, it may represent a reactive process.[2]

Most lesions are solitary, small, sharply demarcated, and uniform in color. Although they may range in size, it is rare for an oral melanotic macule to present as a larger than 1 cm lesion[3] (**Fig. 1**). The average age of affected patients is around 43 years with women more likely to present with these lesions when compared with men.[1]

To rule out malignant melanoma, a biopsy is required.[3] Histopathologically, these lesions will show an increase in melanin in the parabasilar layers of the epithelium without a concomitant increase in the number of melanocytes. On confirmation of diagnosis, no further treatment is necessary. Macules do not exhibit any malignant potential and the prognosis is excellent.[3]

MELANOCYTIC NEVUS

A nevus is a developmental or congenital condition originating on the skin or mucosa. The acquired melanocytic nevus (mole) is the most common of these neoplasms when found on the skin; however, they are uncommon in the oral cavity. Melanocytic nevi are benign tumors derived from the neural crest. Although mutations in the BRAF or NRAS oncogenes are frequent in cutaneous nevi, these mutations may not be associated with nevi of the oral cavity.[4,5]

Clinically, oral melanocytic nevi most commonly are found on the hard palate, followed by the buccal mucosa and vermilion border. These lesions typically are around 0.5 cm in greatest diameter, with approximately 9% presenting as a lesion larger than 1.0 cm. The nevi may present with brown, blue, or black pigmentation, although approximately 15% to 22% are amelanotic[5,6] (**Figs. 2** and **3**). Patients are usually aged older than 30 years at first diagnosis, and women are more commonly affected than men. Caucasians are the most commonly affected group. In the oral cavity, the intramucosal nevus is the most commonly encountered melanocytic nevi,

University of Kentucky College of Dentistry, 770 Rose Street, Lexington, KY 40536, USA
* Corresponding author.
E-mail address: ashley.clark.dds@uky.edu

Oral Maxillofacial Surg Clin N Am 35 (2023) 153–158
https://doi.org/10.1016/j.coms.2022.10.008
1042-3699/23/© 2022 Elsevier Inc. All rights reserved.

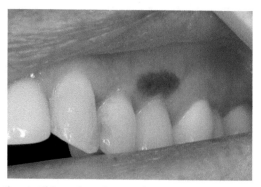

Fig. 1. This melanotic macule presented as a pigmented lesion apical to tooth number 13 on the attached gingiva. (*Courtesy of* Curt Hayes, DDS, Lafayette, CO.)

followed by the blue nevus.[3,4] A biopsy is required to rule out mucosal melanoma.

Histopathologically, the nevus cells may be confined to the epithelium (junctional nevus), found in both the epithelium and superficial lamina propria (compound nevus), or noted entirely in the mucosa (intramucosal nevus). In the blue nevus, melanin-rich melanocytes are noted deep within the mucosa.[4]

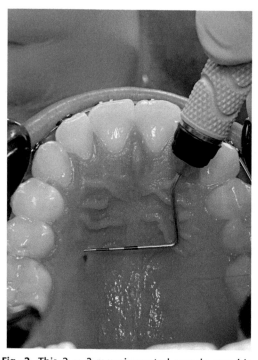

Fig. 2. This 2 × 2 mm-pigmented macule was biopsied; histopathology revealed nevus cells confined to the mucosa. A diagnosis of intramucosal nevus was rendered. (*Courtesy of* Saeid Abbasiyan, DDS, Georgetown, TX.)

The prognosis for oral melanocytic nevi is excellent; malignant transformation into mucosal melanoma has not been well documented.[3]

MELANOACANTHOSIS

Melanoacanthosis, first described as oral melanoacanthoma in 1978 by Tomich, is an uncommon, reactive process, characterized by the distribution of dendritic melanocytes throughout the entire thickness of the epithelium.[7,8] Use of the term melanoacanthosis is currently preferred in order to avoid confusion with the cutaneous lesion, melanoacanthoma of skin. A melanoacanthoma of the skin is considered to be a subtype of seborrheic keratosis and therefore unrelated to the lesion discussed herein.[9]

Melanoacanthosis is found most often in the Black female patient. Clinically, the lesion presents as a solitary, flat or slightly raised, brown macule. The lesion typically exhibits a rapid increase in size before reaching a maximum dimension or approximately 1 to 2 cm within a few weeks.[10] The buccal mucosa is the most frequently involved location, although any oral mucosal surface may be affected. Although typically asymptomatic, pruritus, pain, and a burning sensation have been reported in some cases. Occasionally, patients will report a history of acute or chronic trauma in the area before the lesion appears[3] (**Fig. 4**A, B).

Incisional biopsy is indicated to rule out oral mucosal melanoma especially in cases where rapid increase in size is reported. Histopathologic evaluation will reveal dendritic melanocytes throughout the epithelium in conjunction with spongiosis (**Fig. 4**C). Often the biopsy procedure serves as an impetus for rapid resolution of the pigmentation. Following histopathologic diagnosis, no further intervention is required; the prognosis is excellent.[3,11]

SMOKER'S MELANOSIS

Smoker's melanosis is a nonneoplastic, reactive increase in oral pigmentation in response to irritants in tobacco smoke. It has been hypothesized that the increase in melanin may serve as a protective function.[10,12] This flat, diffuse, brown/black pigmentation typically is noted on the anterior attached gingiva of both arches.[3] Pigmentation tends to appear darker in heavy smokers and has a propensity to occur most often in women, potentially due to a synergistic effect of female sex hormones combined with the effects of smoking. The clinician may make the diagnosis with correlation of smoking history and clinical presentation; staining of the dentition may also serve as a helpful

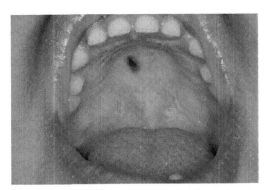

Fig. 3. A 15-year-old male patient presented with a darkly pigmented lesion measuring approximately 1.0 × 0.5 cm on the hard palate. Biopsy proved the diagnosis to be a compound melanocytic nevus. (*Courtesy of* Indraneel Bhattacharyya, DDS, MSD, Gainesville, FL.)

clue to the diagnosis.[10,11] No treatment is necessary, although it is prudent to counsel the patient on smoking cessation, if amenable. It has been reported that the pigmentation dissipates 6 to 36 months after cessation.[10,12]

DRUG-RELATED DISCOLORATIONS OF THE ORAL MUCOSA

There are numerous medications that may be responsible for discoloration of the oral mucosa via multiple pathways including direct incorporation into the tissue or by inducing melanin production.[3,13] Drugs including minocycline, antimalarials, oral contraceptives, chemotherapeutics, zidovudine , ketoconazole, and clofazimine have all been implicated.[3,11,13,14]

Clinically, these pigmented lesions may vary based on the drug causing the reaction. For example, antimalarial drugs tend to affect only the hard palate, while minocycline can lead to a

bluish-black discoloration of the maxilla and mandible leading to dark-appearing gingivae.[13,15] Minocycline may also lead to hyperpigmentation of the oral mucosa due to increase in melanin production.[13] Other drugs may cause diffuse, brown pigmentation of any mucosal surface. The gingivae and buccal mucosa are the most frequently affected sites and it may mimic physiologic pigmentation.[3,10]

A biopsy is only considered for drug-related discolorations of the oral mucosa if a definitive clinical correlation with medication use cannot be established. Microscopically, an increase in melanin may be noted in the parabasilar layers or granules of melanin may be seen in the superficial lamina propria.[3,13] If the medication is discontinued, the discoloration may fade. However, no further action is warranted after appropriate diagnosis.[3]

ADDISON DISEASE

Hypoadrenocorticism, or Addison disease, may lead to diffuse pigmentation of the oral cavity. It has been reported this discoloration affects approximately 92% of patients affected by Addison disease.[13,16] In fact, hyperpigmentation of mucous membrane and cutaneous surfaces is one of the first signs of Addison disease.[3]

Addison disease is a result of an adrenal cortex disorder that results in insufficient levels of glucocorticoid and mineralocorticoid.[17] Increased adrenocorticotropic hormone is secreted in response to low corticosteroid levels. When this occurs, an increase in α-melanocyte-stimulating hormone occurs, leading to melanogenesis and hyperpigmentation.[3,14,18] Autoimmune adrenalitis is the most common cause of Addison disease, although other syndromes, autoimmune conditions, and infections may also lead to disease development.[17]

In addition to the hyperpigmentation, Addison disease is characterized by a slow progression of

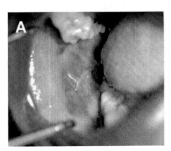
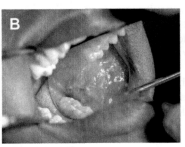
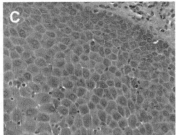

Fig. 4. (*A*) and (*B*) A 36-year-old woman with a chief complaint of bilateral pigmented lesions of the buccal mucosa, which were rapidly increasing in size during the last 1 to 2 months. This patient had similar lesions of the hard palate and lower lip. (*C*) A high-power view of dendritic melanocytes noted throughout the epithelium in oral melanoacanthosis; these are typically only noted in the basilar layers. (*Courtesy of* [*A, B*] Indraneel Bhattacharyya, DDS, MSD, Gainesville, FL.)

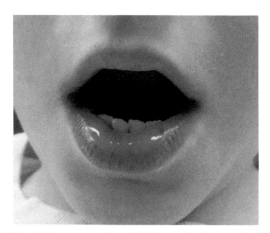

Fig. 5. Numerous pigmented macules in a patient with Peutz-Jeghers syndrome. (*Courtesy of* Sarah Stuart, DDS, Houston, TX.)

nonspecific symptoms, including fatigue, weight loss, nausea, and vomiting. Patients may also experience hyponatremia and hyperkalemia. In around 50% of patients, the disease presents with an adrenal crisis, which is a life-threating condition delineated by shock and severe dehydration.[17]

In the oral cavity, patients with Addison disease may present with generalized macules of hyperpigmentation. The mucous membranes of the oral cavity often are affected before cutaneous involvement occurs. The differential diagnosis includes physiologic pigmentation, although the onset will be acute in a patient with Addison disease.[11,13]

When a health-care provider suspects Addison disease, referral to the patient's primary care physician is warranted; the patient may then be referred to an endocrinologist for diagnosis. Addison disease typically is managed by replacing the glucocorticoid and mineralocorticoid hormones with hydrocortisone and fludrocortisone, respectively. Those with primary adrenal insufficiency also may be prescribed for daily dose of dehydroepiandrosterone. If there is a specific cause, such as infection, the underlying etiology also must be addressed.

Although patients should double their daily dose of glucocorticoid when under increased stress, it is not necessary to increase glucocorticoids for simple dental procedures.[17]

PEUTZ-JEGHERS SYNDROME

Peutz-Jeghers syndrome is an autosomal dominant disease caused by a mutation of the STK11/ LKB1 tumor suppressor gene.[3,13] The syndrome is characterized by hamartomas of the intestine and an increased risk for malignancies. Intussusception of the bowel and/or obstruction may occur in some patients.[13]

Patients with this condition may present with numerous macules of hyperpigmentation on and around the lips during childhood (**Fig. 5**). These areas of hyperpigmentation resemble freckles but do not darken with sun exposure. Pigmentation may also occur intraorally; if so, it is most commonly noted on the buccal mucosa.[3,13]

Once identified, the patient should be referred to their primary care physician or gastroenterologist for further testing and management. Patients diagnosed with Peutz-Jeghers syndrome are treated for intussusception and/or bowel obstruction if necessary. They are also monitored closely due to their increased risk for malignancy.[13]

MELANOMA

Melanoma presenting in the oral cavity may be primary in origin or a metastatic deposit, typically of cutaneous origin. This is an important distinction to make because treatment modalities and prognosis vary. Both primary oral mucosal and metastatic lesions of cutaneous origin are discussed, with a focus on clinical identification and diagnostic workup.

Primary oral mucosal melanoma is a rare, malignant neoplasm of melanocytes, accounting for only 0.5% of all malignant neoplasms found in the oral cavity.[19,20] It presents within a wide age range of the fourth to eighth decades, with the highest incidence in the sixth decade.[19,21] Significant variation exists in both the clinical and histopathologic features.

Clinically, the presentation may range from benign-appearing lesions, such as a solitary localized macule, to more malignant-appearing lesions with irregular borders or an exophytic surface proliferation. Early mucosal melanoma may mimic a melanotic macule, melanocytic nevus, or amalgam tattoo.[10] Tumors may also present with multiple disseminated pigmented lesions. Rarely, amelanotic lesions have been reported as well. The most commonly affected areas are the hard palate and maxillary gingiva, which account for approximately two-thirds of cases[3,10,11] (**Fig. 6**).

Of all cases of melanoma metastatic to the head and neck area, more than 80% are of cutaneous origin; despite this, only approximately 0.6% to 9.3% of patients with cutaneous melanoma will have metastases to the mucosa of the upper aerodigestive tract. The presence of metastatic melanoma in this region typically indicates

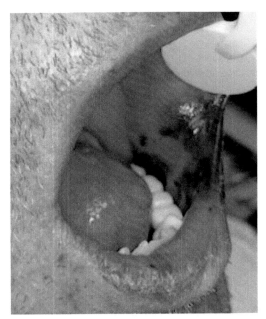

Fig. 6. A patient with oral mucosal melanoma presenting with diffuse, dark pigmentation of the oral cavity, most notably on the left buccal mucosa.

disseminated disease because the most frequent sites of metastasis from cutaneous melanoma are lymph nodes regional to the primary tumor, lung, liver, and brain.[22–24] Similar to their primary counterparts, the clinical presentation of metastatic lesions varies widely, and often mimics benign, reactive lesions, presenting similarly to a pyogenic granuloma. Metastasis typically does not develop until 2 to 7 years after the initial cutaneous lesion. In general, there is no time after which a patient is considered "cured."[23]

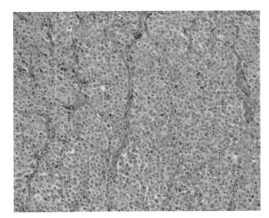

Fig. 7. Lesional cells of an amelanotic melanoma demonstrating sheets and nests of round cells with prominent nucleoli.

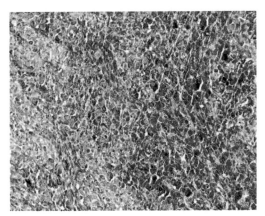

Fig. 8. Prominent pigmentation noted within the lesional cells in a patient with melanoma.

Histopathologically, the neoplastic cells may appear epithelioid, plasmacytoid, or spindle-shaped, with or without pigmentation. A "cherry red" nucleolus is a common feature identified within the nucleus of the neoplastic cells and can be a helpful feature to guide the judicious use of an immunohistochemical panel (**Figs. 7** and **8**).

The histopathologic diagnosis of melanoma of the oral cavity is only the beginning of the definitive diagnostic process for the patient. Systemic evaluation to exclude potential cutaneous primary origin is necessary before designation of an oral lesion as primary mucosal melanoma, as well as to determine extent of metastasis, if applicable.

Although staging criterion is well established for cutaneous melanoma, these tools are not applicable to primary oral mucosal melanoma. A comparison of the 2 finds that oral mucosal melanoma is more lethal when compared with its cutaneous counterpart, with a relatively high recurrence rate even if diagnosed at an early clinical stage. BRAF mutations, common among cutaneous melanomas, may be an option for targeted therapy for cutaneous metastatic lesions. However, these mutations are found in fewer than 10% of oral mucosal melanoma.[23,25] The predominating mutation of oral mucosal melanoma is c-kit, found in up to 30%. RAS mutation is the second most common.[23]

The mainstay of treatment is surgical resection. Adjunctive radiation and chemotherapy are of questionable efficacy but may be used for palliation. Oral mucosal melanoma has an estimated local recurrence rate of up to 85%. The rate of distant metastasis is as high as 50% of cases. As such, prognosis is poor, with 5-year survival rates ranging from 15% to 25% and death often occurring within 2 years of initial diagnosis.[23]

REFERENCES

1. Kaugars GE, Heise AP, Riley WT, et al. Oral mela-notic macules: A review of 353 cases. Oral Surg Oral Med Oral Pathol 1993;76(1):59–61.
2. Buchner A, Merrell PW, Carpenter WM. Relative fre-quency of solitary melanocytic lesions of the oral mucosa. J Oral Pathol Med 2004;33:550–7.
3. Alawi F. Pigmented lesions of the oral cavity: an up-date. Dent Clin North Am 2013;57(4):699–710.
4. Ferreira L, Jham B, Assi R, et al. Oral melanocytic nevi: a clinicopathologic study of 100 cases. Oral Surg Oral Med Oral Pathol Oral Radiol 2015; 120(3):358–67.
5. Freitas DA, Bonan PR, Sousa AA, et al. Intramucosal nevus in the oral cavity. J Contemp Dent Pract 2015; 16(1):74–6.
6. Buchner A, Leider AS, Merrell PW, et al. Melanocytic nevi of the oral mucosa: a clinicopathologic study of 130 cases from northern California. J Oral Pathol Med 1990;19:197–201.
7. Tomich, CE. Oral presentation. (1978) Paper pre-sented at: 32nd Annual Meeting of the American Academy of Oral Pathology. 1978:23–28.
8. Woo S. Oral pathology: A comprehensive atlas and text. Elsevier Health Sciences; 2016. p. 205.
9. Peters S, Mandel L, Perrino M. Oral melanoacan-thoma of the palate: An unusual presentation of an uncommon entity. JAAD Case Rep 2018;4(2):138–9.
10. Neville B, Damm D, Allen C, et al. Oral and maxillo-facial pathology: Fourth edition. St Louis (MO): Elsevier, Inc. 2015, p. 289–92, 349–55, 401–7.
11. Müller S. Melanin-associated pigmented lesions of the oral mucosa: presentation, differential diagnosis, and treatment. Dermatol Ther 2010;23:220–9.
12. Hedin CA, Pindborg JJ, Axéll T. Disappearance of smoker's melanosis after reducing smoking. J Oral Pathol Med 1993;22:228–30.
13. Rosebush MS, Briody AN, Cordell KG. Black and Brown: Non-neoplastic Pigmentation of the Oral Mu-cosa. Head Neck Pathol 2019;13(1):47–55.
14. Granstein RD, Sober AJ. Drug-and heavy metal-induced hyperpigmentation. J Am Acad Dermatol 1981;5:1–18.
15. Lerman MA, Karimbux N, Guze KA, et al. Pigmenta-tion of the hard palate. Oral Surg Oral Med Oral Pathol Oral Radiol Endod 2009;107(1):8–12.
16. Sreeja C, Ramakrishnan K, Vijayalakshmi D, et al. Oral pigmentation: a review. J Pharm Bioallied Sci 2015;7(2):403–8.
17. Chakera AJ, Vaidya B. Addison Disease in Adults: Diagnosis and Management. Am J Med 2010;123: 409–13.
18. Nieman LK, Chanco Turner ML. Addison's disease. Clin Dermatol 2006;24(4):276–80.
19. Bhullar RP, Bhullar A, Vanaki SS, et al. Primary mel-anoma of oral mucosa: A case report and review of literature. Dent Res J 2012;9(3):353–6.
20. Patton LL, Brahim JS, Baker AR. Metastatic malig-nant melanoma of the oral cavity. A retrospective study. Oral Surg Oral Med Oral Pathol 1994;78:51–6.
21. Delgado Azañero WA, Mosqueda Taylor A. A practical method for clinical diagnosis of oral mucosal melanomas. Med Oral 2003;8:348–52.
22. Billings KR, Wang MB, Sercarz JA, et al. Clinical and pathologic distinction between primary and meta-static mucosal melanoma of the head and neck. Otolaryngol Head Neck Surg 1995;112(6):700–6.
23. Wenig B. Atlas of head and neck pathology. Third Edition. St Louis, MO: Elsevier, Inc; 2015. p. 356–8.
24. El-Naggar AK, Chan JK, Grandis JR, et al. WHO classification of head and neck tumours. Lyon: Inter-national Agency for Research on Cancer; 2017.
25. Chapman MD, Hauschild A, Robert C, et al. Improved Survival with Vemurafenib in Melanoma with BRAF V600E Mutation. N Engl J Med 2011; 364:2507–16.

Bacterial Lesions of the Oral Mucosa

Leticia Ferreira Cabido, DDS, MS[a],*, Mário José Romañach, DDS, MSc, PhD[b]

KEYWORDS

- Actinomycosis • Tuberculosis • Syphilis • Scarlet fever • Gonorrhea • Leprosy
- Nonodontogenic bacterial lesions • Oral bacterial lesions

KEY POINTS

- Most nonodontogenic bacterial lesions are highly infectious; therefore, early diagnosis and treatment are of the utmost importance.
- These lesions may clinically and microscopically mimic other oral diseases, which complicate early diagnosis.
- Syphilis and gonorrhea cases are increasing in the United States; hence, it is prudent that clinicians be familiar with their potential oral manifestations.
- Although most of the oral bacterial diseases are easily treatable, delay in the diagnosis can lead to life-threatening complications.

INTRODUCTION

Nonodontogenic bacterial infections of the oral cavity are not a common finding in the United States. Nevertheless, there has been an increase in the prevalence of certain bacterial sexually transmitted diseases, such as syphilis and gonorrhea, and conditions such as tuberculosis (TB) still pose a serious threat to certain segments of the population. Finally, given the uncommon nature and the widespread clinical presentation and pathophysiology of these diseases, diagnosis is often delayed, resulting in more clinically significant disease and potential contamination of individuals. Thus, it is prudent that clinicians be familiar with these uncommon but potentially serious infectious diseases, so treatment can be instituted promptly.

Actinomycosis

Actinomycosis is a suppurative infection of filamentous, anaerobic bacterial species of the genus *Actinomyces*. Actinomycetes are gram-positive, pigment-producing bacilli that are considered normal saprophytic components of the oral flora, mainly from tonsillar crypts (forming concretions plugs), dental plaque, carious dentin, bone sequestra, salivary calculi, gingival sulci, and periodontal pockets. These bacteria are often isolated with other normal commensals (polymicrobial infection), reinforcing the hypothesis that other organisms may create favorable conditions (oxygen tension reduction and host defenses inhibition) to support their continued growth.

Actinomycosis is often underreported and misdiagnosed. The low potential of invasiveness and virulence contributes to the lack of incidence data. Cervicofacial actinomycosis may mimic other conditions, making diagnosis very difficult. Culture is usually negative due to the anaerobic nature of the organism, the prolonged incubation period, and the empirical use of many antibiotics, to which Actinomyces are highly sensitive.[1-4] The invasion of oral tissues by actinomycetes is attributed to loss of integrity and chronic inflammation not only from previous trauma but also from fractures, surgery, tooth extraction, endodontic

[a] Department of Diagnosis and Oral Health, University of Louisville School of Dentistry 501 South Preston St. Louisville, KY 40202, USA; [b] Department of Oral Diagnosis and Pathology, School of Dentistry, Universidade Federal do Rio de Janeiro (UFRJ), Brazil
* Corresponding author.
E-mail address: leticia.cabido@louisville.edu

Oral Maxillofacial Surg Clin N Am 35 (2023) 159–173
https://doi.org/10.1016/j.coms.2022.10.009
1042-3699/23/© 2022 Published by Elsevier Inc.

treatment, sinusitis, periodontal disease, or peri-apical infection.[1–3]

Clinical Findings

- Cervicofacial actinomycosis accounts for more than half of the cases[2–4]
  - *Actinomyces israelii* and *Actinomyces gerencseriae* are responsible for 70% of cases
  - Chronic hard swelling in the mandible and/or the neck
    - "Wooden" indurated fibrosis (lumpy jaw) in 60% of cases
  - Associated soft tissue abscess with minimal pain and mild fever
  - Sinus tracts draining pus containing sulfur granules
    - Dark red to purple overlying skin of non-healing sinus tracts
- Young healthy adults: men > women
- Jaw involvement
  - Mandible > maxilla (4:1)
  - Association with osteomyelitis, and persistent periapical inflammatory lesions (**Fig. 1**)
- Other sites may be involved
  - Larynx, hypopharynx, lacrimal and salivary glands, oral mucosa (tongue)[1]
- Systemic manifestations: Fever, chills, and weight loss

Differential Diagnosis

- Other bacterial infections, TB, nocardiosis, cyst, and malignancy[4]

Diagnostic Modalities

- Gram staining of pus and/or microscopic evaluation[4]
- Molecular techniques have improved organism identification
  - 16S ribosomal RNA (rRNA) sequencing and polymerase chain reaction (PCR)

Imaging

- Evaluation of bone involvement, disease extent, and treatment
  - Computed tomography, MRI, and ultrasonography[3,4]

Pathology

- The sulfur granules are round gritty colonies of *Actinomyces* observed in vivo
  - Whitish gray, yellow, brownish green, or green in color
  - There is no evidence that the granules contain sulfur

- They are not pathognomonic (also produced by other types of bacteria)
- It offers bacteria protection against immune cells
- Identified histologically but frequently lost during tissue handling and processing
- Masses of club-shaped filaments arranged in radiating rosette pattern (**Fig. 2**)
  - Surrounded by neutrophils
  - Mineralized and cemented by host calcium phosphate
- Granulomatous inflammation with central necrosis may be present
  - Lymphocytes, plasma cells, epithelioid cells, histiocytes, and giant cells
- The periphery of the lesion can be fibrotic and avascular[2,3,5]

Therapeutic Options

- Surgical removal of infected tissue and appropriate antibiotic therapy
  - Abscess drainage, removal of necrotic bone, dental extraction, and/or excision of sinus tracts
- Penicillin G or amoxicillin
  - Severe (deep and chronic) cases—intravenous amoxicillin (up to 200 mg/kg/d) or penicillin G (up to 24 MIU/d) followed by oral treatment
  - Prolonged treatment of up to 6 to 12 months is questionable
  - Several investigators advocate that localized acute actinomycotic infections (eg, periapical and pericoronal actinomycosis) be treated more conservatively (surgical removal of infected tissue) and that antibiotics be reserved for cases in which invasion of surrounding structures and spread through the soft tissues is seen
- Long-term follow-up recommended
- Good prognosis for early treated patients[4,6]

Tuberculosis

TB is a chronic communicable disease caused by *Mycobacterium tuberculosis*. The disease remains one of the most serious infectious diseases in the world and until before the coronavirus (COVID-19) pandemic, it represented the leading cause of death from a single infectious agent.[7]

According to the WHO, an estimated 9.9 million people became ill with TB worldwide in 2020, with approximately 1.5 million deaths reported.[7] In contrast, for the year of 2020, the United States reported only 7174 cases of TB and an incidence rate of only 2.2 cases per 100,000 persons. Although US rates are low and have been declining

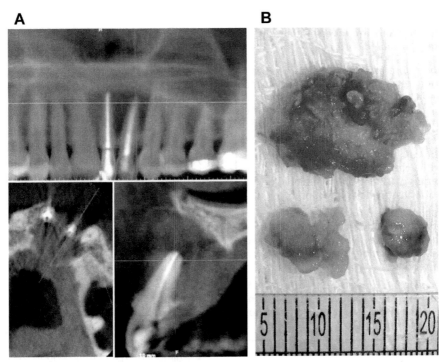

Fig. 1. (*A*) A persistent periapical lesion after endodontic treatment of upper incisors of an adult patient. (*B*) The gross appearance of the sample biopsied included a round grayish-colored soft fragment, measuring 5 mm, which consisted of colonies of *Actinomyces* (lower right).

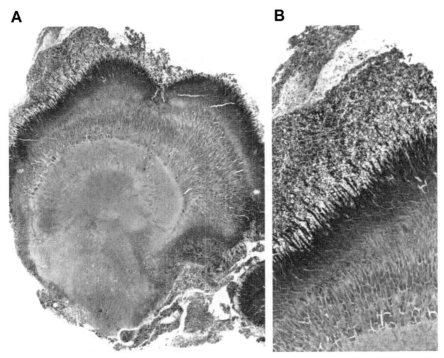

Fig. 2. Typical radiating architecture of partially mineralized, club-shaped filaments of *Actinomyces* surrounded by neutrophils (hematoxylin and eosin, *A*, 100× and *B*, 400×).

Box 1
Important definitions for understanding the pathogenesis of tuberculosis

Latent tuberculosis infection: It is characterized by the presence of immunologic sensitivity to mycobacterial antigen (as determined by a tuberculin skin test or an interferon-γ release assay) in the absence of the clinical symptoms of disease.[15]

Active tuberculosis or tuberculosis disease: It is diagnosed in patients who have clinical signs and symptoms of TB and show microbiological evidence of *M tuberculosis* infection.[15]

Miliary tuberculosis: It occurs when tubercle bacilli enter the bloodstream and disseminate to all parts of the body, where they grow and cause disease in multiple sites. This condition is rare but serious.[13]

Oral tuberculosis: It is a rare form of extrapulmonary TB, which affects only 0.1% to 5% of individuals with the disease. It may or may not coexist with pulmonary TB.[16]

for the past several years, the disease still disproportionately affects certain segments of the population such as racial and ethnic minorities, foreign-born persons, those living in crowded living situations, and suffering from underlying medical conditions (eg, diabetes mellitus and infection with human immunodeficiency virus [HIV]).[8,9]

M tuberculosis is contracted by inhalation of airborne microorganisms that are generated by individuals with active TB.[10] Primary TB occurs in previously unexposed people, almost always involves the lungs, produces only mild symptoms, and generally goes undiagnosed. Most patients exposed to the bacterium develop a strong cell-mediated immune response that stops the progression of the infection.[11] When this happens, the initial lung and nodal lesions of primary TB, undergo progressive inspissation, hardening, encapsulation, often followed by radiologically detectable calcification.[11,12] Although the lesion "heals," some bacteria may remain dormant in these fibrocalcific nodules.[12] Latent tuberculosis infection (LTBI) is the term used when the host defenses can contain *M tuberculosis* microorganisms but the organisms still maintain the capacity to replicate and cause disease in the future (**Box 1**).[13,14]

Only in a very small proportion of patients, usually young children and the immunocompromised, the initial infection is not controlled by the immune response and the patient progresses rapidly to active TB. Dissemination of bacilli may occur through the lung parenchyma, resulting in extensive pulmonary lesions and lymphohematogenous spread. Widespread infection with multiple organ involvement is called miliary TB.[3,12,13] More commonly, however, TB disease develops months to years after the initial infection, due to a reactivation of LTBI. This reactivation is usually the result of a weakened immune system, and some individuals are at an increased risk of disease reactivation (**Box 2**).[9,13]

Although TB primarily affects the lungs, it can be seen in other sites such as lymph nodes, pleura, genitourinary tract, and the oral cavity. Oral lesions can occur either in the primary or secondary forms of TB. The lesions are believed to be the result of autoinoculation by *M tuberculosis* bacilli in the sputum, or through hematogenous or lymphatic spread.[17]

Clinical Findings

- Unexplained weight loss, low grade fever, night sweats, anorexia, and fatigue[11,13]
- Pulmonary TB: chronic cough, pleuritic pain, and hemoptysis[11]
- Oral TB
  - Men > women[18,19]
  - Fourth and fifth decades of life[16,18,19]
  - Typically presents as soft tissue lesions but one-fourth of cases are intraosseous[19]
  - Soft tissue lesions
    - Predilection for tongue, followed by buccal mucosa, gingiva, palate, and lips[18,19]

Box 2
Persons at increased risk for progression of latent tuberculosis infection to tuberculosis disease

[a]Persons infected with HIV

Children aged younger than 5 years

Persons recently infected with *M tuberculosis* (within the past 2 years)

Persons who are receiving immunosuppressive therapy such as tumor necrosis factor-alpha antagonists, corticosteroids, or immunosuppressive drug therapy following organ transplantation

Persons with diabetes mellitus

Cigarette smokers and persons who abuse drugs and/or alcohol

[a]Considered the strongest known risk factor for progression to TB disease.

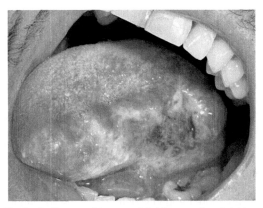

Fig. 3. A 40-year-old man with history of weight loss (22 lbs) and persistent cough for the last 4 months. (A) The patient presented a painful ulcer involving the left border of the tongue of 1-month duration as an oral manifestation of tuberculosis. (*Courtesy of Rafaela França, DDS, Rio de Janeiro, BR.*)

- Ulceration, typically described as indurated, with ill-defined margins and a hard necrotic base[16,19] (**Fig. 3**)
- Swelling, nodules, fissures, and granulation tissue-like or granular lesions have been reported[18,19]
  - Intraosseous lesions:
    - Mandible far more often affected than maxilla[18,19]
    - Radiolucent, destructive bony swellings[18,19]
      - Symptoms of tenderness, pain or burning, may be present[19]
      - Secondary oral TB is more common than primary oral TB and tends to affect middle-aged and elderly patients[17]
      - Primary oral TB typically occurs in children and adolescents and presents as an asymptomatic ulcer with concomitant enlargement of cervical lymph nodes[17]
      - Although persons with extrapulmonary TB are usually not infectious, lesions of oral cavity or larynx should be considered infectious[13]
- Neck TB
  - Cervical lymph nodes are more commonly affected by TB than the oral cavity with the submental and submandibular lymph nodes affected most often[16,20,21]
  - Involvement of major salivary glands is also possible
  - Lymph node involvement most commonly presents as a localized mass, resulting from infection of intracapsular or pericapsular lymph nodes[21]

- May present as parenchymatous fistula/sinus tracts or an abscess[21] (**Fig. 4**)

Differential diagnosis

- Most cases of oral TB have been clinically mistaken for a malignant process, especially squamous cell carcinoma[16,19]

Diagnostic Modalities

- Two methods available in the United States for the detection of *M tuberculosis* infection:
  - TB blood tests (interferon-gamma release assays [IGRAs])
    - QuantiFERON-TB Gold Plus (QFT-Plus)
    - T-SPOT.TB test (T-Spot)
  - Mantoux tuberculin skin test
- These tests cannot distinguish LTBI from active TB disease
- Acid-fast stains and culture of infected sputum or tissue must be used to confirm the diagnosis of active disease
- Nuclei acid amplification (NAA) tests can be used to rapidly identify the microorganisms in the specimen. It can detect *M tuberculosis* DNA in just hours, compared with a week or more for the detection of the organism in culture
  - Allows earlier detection of drug resistance when certain NAAs are used (eg, Gene Xpert)
- A posterior-anterior radiograph of the chest is mandatory for all cases suspicious for TB[13,17]
- Oral TB:
  - A biopsy of the oral ulcer is of utmost importance to confirm oral TB and rule out other important lesions in the differential diagnosis such as a carcinoma
    - The microscopic presence of caseous granulomas in an oral biopsy is not diagnostic of TB but will prompt the pathologist to order Ziehl-Neelsen (ZN) or other acid-fast stains to aid in the identification of the mycobacteria
    - The ZN sensitivity can be low, thus a negative result does not rule out the possibility of TB
    - Molecular tests are more sensitive and may enhance the diagnosis
    - Even if the microorganism is detected in the biopsy specimen, identification of the organism by culture is recommended

Pathology

- Microscopically, TB is characterized by the presence of granulomas which are collections

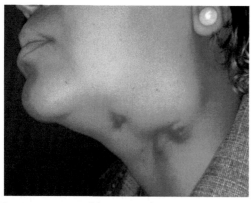

Fig. 4. A 47-year-old woman presents with neck fistulas secondary to TB involvement of cervical lymph nodes. (*Courtesy of* Fernando Lima, DDS, Rio de Janeiro, BR.)

of giant cells and epithelioid histiocytes and which may show central caseous necrosis[19]
- Tiny, rod-shaped, acid-fast bacilli may be identified with ZN or Kinyoun stain[2] (**Fig. 5**)

Therapeutic Options

- TB disease is generally treated for 6 months
  - Two phases: the intensive phase and the continuation phase
    - Intensive phase: A 2-month treatment regimen that includes the 4 first-line anti-TB drugs: isoniazid, rifampin, ethambutol, and pyrazinamide
    - Continuation phase: An additional 4 months of treatment, which include 2 drugs, usually isoniazid and rifampin[13]
- Several treatments are available for persons with LTBI. The CDC currently recommends a rifamycin-based, 3-month or 4-month treatment regimen[13]

Syphilis

Syphilis is an infectious, sexually transmitted disease caused by the spirochete bacterium *Treponema pallidum*. Syphilis is reemerging in several countries.[22] In the United States, the national rate of reported cases of primary and secondary (P&S) syphilis has increased almost every year since 2001, increasing 6.8% during 2019 to 2020. Men account for most cases of syphilis, with most of those cases occurring in men who have sex with men (MSM). MSM are disproportionately affected by syphilis, accounting for a majority (53%) of all male P&S syphilis cases in 2020. However, in recent years, the increases in P&S syphilis have slowed among MSM. In contrast,

although rates of P&S syphilis are lower in women, rates have increased in recent years, increasing 21% during 2019 to 2020 and 147% during 2016 to 2020.[23]

The main mode of transmission is through sexual contact (acquired syphilis) but it can also be transmitted vertically by transplacental spread (congenital syphilis).[3] Once acquired, syphilis evolves through a series of 4 overlapping stages: primary, secondary, latent, and tertiary. Each stage is characterized by specific clinical findings and levels of infectivity.[24]

Oral mucosal lesions may be seen in all stages but are more frequently detected in the secondary stage, when they may represent the first clinical manifestation of this serious contagious disease.[25] Unfortunately, oral manifestations of syphilis are often difficult to diagnose, and this disease has been described as "the great imitator" because it commonly mimics many different diseases.

Clinical Findings

- Primary syphilis
  - Characterized by the highly contagious chancre, which develops at the site of inoculation
    - Appears 3 to 90 days after exposure and usually starts as a papule that may evolve into an indurated, painless, nonpurulent ulcer with a clean base and a sharply marginated border
  - Oral primary syphilis
    - Most extragenital chancres (40%–75%) are found in the oral cavity, with lesions typically occurring on the upper or lower lip or the tongue[22]
    - Typically a painless, clean-based ulcer.[2]
  - Typically followed 7 to 10 days later by painless regional lymphadenopathy and chancre shows regression even without any treatment within 2 to 8 weeks[25]
  - If the patient is not treated, the microorganisms will proliferate and then disseminate throughout the body via hematogenous spread, setting the stage for the secondary phase[22,25]
- Secondary syphilis
  - Appears 2 to 12 weeks after exposure to the microorganism and may develop during or after regression of the chancre[22,25]
  - Constitutional symptoms, such as malaise, sore throat, headache, weight loss, low-grade fever, and generalized lymphadenopathy, are usually present[22]
  - The most common presentation is the presence of a skin rash characterized by

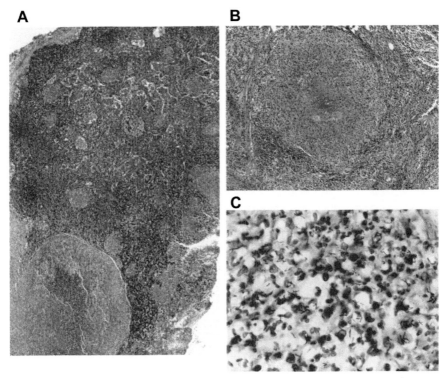

Fig. 5. (*A, B*) Granulomas containing central necrosis affecting a lymph node of a patient with tuberculosis. (*C*) Acid-fast stain revealed numerous mycobacterial organisms presenting as red, rod-shaped bacilli (hematoxylin and eosin, *A*, 50× and *B*, 100×; Ziehl-Neelsen, *C*, 400×).

nonpruritic pink or red macules or papules, symmetrically distributed on the palms, soles, flanks, and arms[26] (**Fig. 6**)
- ○ Skin lesions may mimic lichen planus, eczema, psoriasis, pityriasis, and drug eruptions[22]
- ○ Alopecia may be seen.[22]
- ○ Oral secondary syphilis
  - Most characteristic finding is the highly contagious and painful mucous patches
    - multiple, painful, slightly elevated, whitish plaques or ulcerations[3] (**Fig. 7**)
    - when patches become confluent, a serpiginous or snail track appearance is seen[2,3]
    - tongue, lip, buccal mucosa, and palate[2]
- ○ Raised papillary lesions known as condylomata lata may be seen in the genital or anal areas, and less commonly in oral mucosa[2,22]
- ○ This stage lasts for weeks, or months and relapses may occur[3]
- Latent syphilis
  - ○ After the secondary phase, patient is asymptomatic, and disease is only detectable through serologic testing.[3,25]
  - ○ May last 1 to 30 years[3]

- Tertiary syphilis
  - ○ The most serious stage; life-threatening neurologic (eg, sensory deficits, tabes dorsalis, psychosis) and cardiovascular complications (eg, ascending aortitis, aneurysm) may develop
  - ○ Develops in one-third of untreated patients[22]
  - ○ Transmission is unlikely[3]
  - ○ Nodular, indurated, or ulcerated lesion termed gumma may involve skin, liver, bones, or any other organ[22,25]
  - ○ Oral tertiary syphilis
    - Destructive gummas, which tend to be seen in the hard palate and tongue
      - Bone destruction, palatal perforation, oro-nasal fistula, and extensive osteonecrosis may be seen[3,25]
      - Tongue lesions can produce diffuse atrophy (luetic glossitis) or a large lobulated or irregular appearance of the tongue (interstitial glossitis)[24]

Differential Diagnosis

- Oral lesions of secondary syphilis can be diverse and nonspecific, often clinically mimicking other diseases.

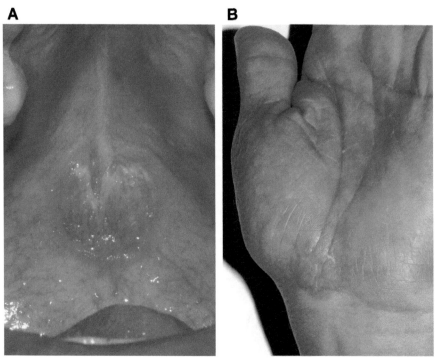

Fig. 6. A 34-year-old man presenting with (*A*) a red and white plaque located in the soft palate as an oral manifestation of secondary syphilis. (*B*) Reddish macules were observed on his palms. (*Courtesy of* Michelle Agostini, DDS, Rio de Janeiro, BR.)

- Chancre may resemble a squamous cell carcinoma, traumatic ulceration, deep fungal infection (eg, histoplasmosis, blastomycosis), or TB.[24]
- Mucous patches may clinically resemble leukoplakia, hyperkeratosis, oral hairy leukoplakia (see **Fig. 7**), or conditions that cause multifocal ulcerations with pseudomembranes such as atypical/major aphthous ulcerations, erosive lichen planus, erythema multiforme, pemphigus vulgaris, geographic tongue, Crohn disease, and granulomatosis with polyangiitis.[3,24]

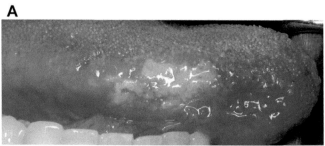

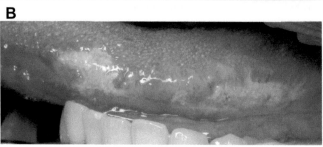

Fig. 7. A 58-year-old woman presenting with bilateral, painful whitish plaques affecting the lateral border of the tongue (*A, B*), which represented mucous patches of secondary syphilis. (*Courtesy of* Eric Rabey, DDS, Fresno, CA.)

- Condylomata lata may be mistaken for squamous papilloma and condyloma acuminatum.

Diagnostic Modalities

- Diagnosis of oral lesions in patients not known to be infected with *T pallidum* begins with a biopsy
  - Confirmation through serologic testing should follow immediately
    - Venereal Disease Research Laboratory
    - Rapid plasma reagin
    - *T pallidum* particle agglutination assay
    - Fluorescent treponemal antibody absorption
    - These tests are accurate for diagnosis and following a patient's response to treatment

Pathology

- Features are relatively nonspecific and may mimic inflammatory lesions
- Clinical correlation is of utmost importance for the pathologist to be able to suspect syphilis and order the appropriate tests
- The lesion typically reveals a dense plasmacytic/lymphocytic infiltrate in the superficial lamina propria and occasionally in the deeper stroma (**Fig. 8**)
- Infiltrate tends to surround blood vessels and nerves
- Epithelium shows ulceration or hyperplasia with extensive exocytosis of inflammatory cells[2,24]
- Silver staining, immunofluorescent, or immunohistochemical techniques allow the identification of the spirochetes[22,24] (**Fig. 9**).

Therapeutic Options

- Recommended treatment of P&S syphilis among adults is benzathine penicillin G, 2.4 million units IM in a single dose.[27]
- For those who are allergic to penicillin, prescriptions of doxycycline 100 mg orally twice daily for 14 days or tetracycline (500 mg 4 times daily for 14 days) can be effective.[27]

Scarlet Fever

Scarlet fever (SF) is a systemic condition caused by group A, β-hemolytic streptococci. It typically begins as a streptococcal pharyngitis (strep throat) but less commonly it can follow group A streptococcal pyoderma or wound infections.[28] The streptococci elaborate an erythrogenic toxin that attacks the blood vessels. Patients who do not elaborate antitoxin antibodies are susceptible to this condition. SF is characterized by a skin rash, lingual mucosal changes, and fever.[2]

Group A streptococcal infection, including SF, are typically spread through direct contact with the saliva or nasal secretions from an infected person. The incubation period of SF is approximately 2 to 5 days.[28]

Clinical Findings

- Typically affects children aged between 5 and 15 years; rare in children aged younger than 3 years[28]
- Affected patients typically have a fever and sore throat 1 to 2 days before developing a rash[29]
  - Begins on the upper part of the trunk and travels distally, sparing the soles and hands[3,29]
  - Characterized by confluent, erythematous macules that blanch under pressure, resembling a sunburn[29]
  - Small, pinhead papules, which are normal in color, project through the erythematous macules, giving the skin a characteristic sandpaper feel or the appearance of "sunburn with goose pimples"[2,3]
  - The cheeks may seem flushed with a characteristic circumoral pallor[3]
  - In skinfolds and areas of pressure, an erythematous linear eruption, which may seem petechial or mildly hemorrhagic (Pastia lines) may be seen[3,29]
  - Rash persists for approximately a week and is followed by desquamation of the skin, which can last several weeks[28,29]
- Intraoral findings
  - White tongue coating may initially be noted through which only the fungiform papillae is seen (white strawberry tongue); by the fourth or fifth day, the white coating desquamates, exposing an erythematous dorsal tongue with hyperplastic fungiform papillae (red strawberry tongue)[2] (**Fig.10**).
  - Tonsils, soft palate, and pharynx may seem red and edematous; the tonsillar crypts may contain yellowish exudate.[2]
  - Petechiae may be seen on the soft palate.[2]
- Cervical lymphadenopathy, headache, fatigue, nausea, vomiting, and myalgias may be present[3]

Differential Diagnosis

- Various viral diseases that can cause acute pharyngitis with a viral exanthema

A

B

C

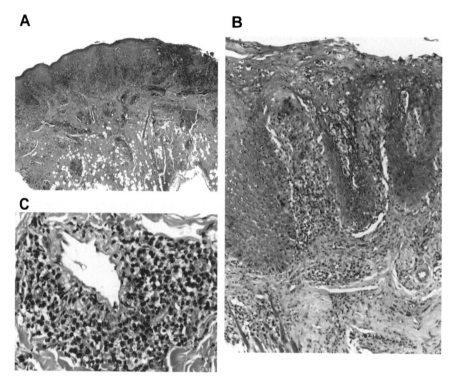

Fig. 8. Microscopic features of syphilis include (*A*) a subepithelial and perivascular chronic inflammatory infiltrate. (*B*) The hyperplastic epithelium exhibits extensive neutrophilic exocytosis, and (*C*) there are a predominance of plasma cells around the blood vessels in the connective tissue (Hematoxylin and eosin, *A*, 25×; *B* and *C*, 100×).

Diagnostic Modalities

- Rapid antigen detection test (RADT) or throat culture
  - RADT has high specificity for group A *Streptococcus* but varying sensitives.
  - Throat culture is gold standard; clinicians should follow-up a negative RADT in a child with characteristic symptoms of SF with a throat culture.

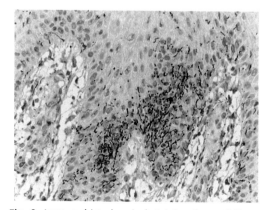

Fig. 9. Immunohistochemical staining for anti-*Treponema pallidum* revealed many spirochetes observed within the epithelium and superficial lamina propria.

Therapeutic Options

- Penicillin or amoxicillin is the antibiotic of choice.[28]
- Cephalexin, cefadroxil, clindamycin, or azithromycin for those allergic to penicillin.
- Prompt treatment after a positive RADT or throat culture is important to prevent rare complications such as peritonsillar or retropharyngeal abscess, sinusitis, pneumonia, acute rheumatic fever, and glomerulonephritis.[2,28]

Gonorrhea

Gonorrhea is the second most reported bacterial communicable infection in United States, with estimated 1,568,000 new cases per year, women being affected slightly more than men. Urethral gonorrhea infections in men, when treated early, do not cause major sequelae but often contribute to their transmission. Among women, gonococcal infections do not produce recognizable symptoms until the occurrence of complications such as pelvic inflammatory disease (PID), which can result in tubal scarring, infertility, or ectopic pregnancy. The treatment of gonorrhea is of significant public health concern because it may be complicated

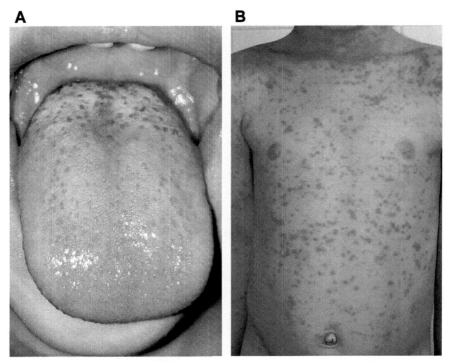

Fig. 10. A 5-year-old boy with (*A*) a strawberry tongue and history of fever and sore throat 5 days before developing (*B*) a skin rash in the trunk. (*Courtesy of* Aline Corrêa Abrahão, DDS, Rio de Janeiro, BR.)

by the ability of *Neisseria gonorrhoeae* to develop antimicrobial resistance.[3,30]

Gonorrhea is a sexually transmitted infection (STI) caused by *N gonorrhoeae*.[2,3] It is usually transmitted during vaginal intercourse, from infected men to women aged between 15 and 30 years, with higher prevalence among sexually active young adults from low-income countries, as well as sexual and gender minorities, racial/ethnic minorities, indigenous communities, and sex workers.[31]

Clinical Findings

- Mildly symptomatic urethritis in men: dysuria and clear to mucopurulent discharge[2,3]
- Most women remain asymptomatic but cervicitis may cause dysuria, increased purulent vaginal discharge, intermenstrual bleeding, and genital itching
  - Involvement of ovarian tubes and uterus may lead to PID, and long-term reproductive complications such as infertility or ectopic pregnancies
- Anal sex may result in painful proctitis with purulent discharge and bleeding
- Newborns of asymptomatic women with gonorrhea are at risk of blindness due to gonococcal ophthalmia neonatorum, whereas autoinoculation of gonococcus may cause acute purulent conjunctivitis and corneal ulceration in adults

- Disseminated gonococcal infection is observed in 0.5% to 3% of untreated individuals[2,3]
  - Myalgia, migratory polyarthritis, and skin rash with hemorrhagic pustules on the extremities
  - Fever, endocarditis, pericarditis, meningitis, and aphthous-like ulceration of the soft palate and oropharynx
  - Occasional association with dermatitis-tenosynovitis syndrome and septic arthritis syndrome
- Oropharyngeal gonorrhea most commonly affects the pharynx, tonsils, and uvula
  - Women or men who have sex with men and likely a result of fellatio, gonococcal septicemia, kissing, or cunnilingus[32]
  - Erythematous edema of oropharynx or tonsils (gonococcal tonsillitis less common than pharyngitis)
  - Mild-to-moderate sore throat, occasionally with small pustules
  - Occasionally associated with concomitant urethritis, cervicitis, or proctitis
- Oral gonorrhea
  - Uncommon; it usually appears in the first week after the sexual contact[2]

○ Infected areas may seem erythematous, pustular, erosive, or ulcerated covered by a white pseudomembrane
○ Submandibular lymphadenopathy
○ Rare secondary infection of the parotid glands

Differential Diagnosis

• May acute necrotizing ulcerative gingivitis/periodontitis (usually lacks the typical fetor oris, aphthous stomatitis, oral lichen planus, erythema multiforme, and primary herpetic gingivostomatitis

Diagnostic Modalities

• Microscopy, culture of endocervical swabs, or nucleic acid amplification tests[30,33]

Therapeutic Options

• Recently, *N gonorrhoeae* has shown a high prevalence of strains resistant to treatment using most available antimicrobials
• Currently a single dose of ceftriaxone 500 mg intramuscularly is recommended for the treatment of uncomplicated gonococcal infections of the cervix, urethra, rectum, and pharynx among adults and adolescents
• Individuals with gonorrhea should be counseled about the importance of screening their last sexual partners and should be screened for other STIs (eg, coinfection with *Chlamydia trachomatis*)[30]

Leprosy

Leprosy (Hansen disease) is a slowly progressive, nonfatal infectious disease caused by the acid-fast bacillus *Mycobacterium leprae*.[34] It is characterized by a chronic granulomatous inflammation that affects mainly the skin and peripheral nerves. The mechanism of transmission of *M leprae* is still unknown. Leprosy may be classified by clinical presentation or by bacterial index (**Boxes 3 and 4**).

Leprosy is a major public health concern worldwide, being mainly observed in countries with poverty such as India and Brazil, which currently accounts for most of the new cases. Leprosy is the main infectious cause of disability; the permanent crippling physical deformities caused by the disease may lead to significant psychological and social issues. Despite the global prevalence reduction by the implementation of multidrug therapy-based leprosy programs, the prevention, early detection, and appropriate treatment of leprosy remain a significant challenge.[2,3,34]

Diagnostic Symptom Criteria

• Hypopigmented or erythematous skin macules, papules, and nodules with definite loss of sensation
• Thickened or enlarged peripheral nerve with loss of sensation and/or weakness of muscle supplied by the nerve
• Positive acid-fast skin smear or bacilli observed in a skin smear/biopsy[34]

Clinical Findings

• Skin of the face, legs, and buttocks are the most affected sites
• Loss of hair from eyebrows and eyelashes
• Distorted facial appearance (leonine facies) is caused by facial enlargements
• Destructive lesions of the facial bones (facies leprosa) are characterized by
  ○ Atrophy of the anterior maxillary alveolar ridge
    ▪ It may lead to the loss of the incisors
  ○ Atrophy the anterior nasal spine
  ○ Endonasal inflammatory changes
    ▪ Complaints of a stuffy nose, epistaxis, and hyposmia[2,3,35]
• Oral leprosy
  ○ Nonspecific and observed mainly in the lepromatous leprosy (**Fig. 11**)
  ○ Sessile nodules that tend to ulcerate leading to necrosis and fibrosis
  ○ Mainly in the anterior upper gingiva, the palate, and the tonsils/glossopharyngeal arches
  ○ Bleeding or altered sensitivity may be present
  ○ Poor oral conditions secondary to physical disability and depression[36,37]
• Cranial nerve involvement (trigeminal and facial nerves)
  ○ Anesthesia of the orofacial tissues and facial nerve palsies
  ○ Difficulty in mastication, speech, and social relationship[34]

Differential Diagnosis

• Leprosy may mimic a broad list of diseases because of its wide clinical spectrum of dermatologic, neurologic, and oral manifestations.
• Many diseases should be considered in differential diagnosis such as
  ○ allergic reactions, fungal infections, vitiligo, TB, systemic lupus erythematosus, sarcoidosis, mucocutaneous leishmaniasis,

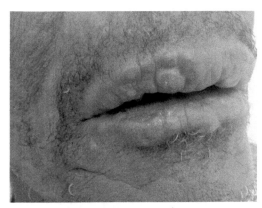

Fig. 11. Asymptomatic lip nodules of lepromatous leprosy of 1-month duration. (*Courtesy of* Wilson Ivo Pinto, DDS, Rio de Janeiro, BR.)

syphilis, diabetes, traumatic lesions, and malignancy.
- Loss of pinprick or light-touch sensation is helpful.
- Loss of sensation or neuropathy may not always be present.[2,3]

Diagnostic Modalities

- Slit skin smear test: bacilloscopy
- Biopsy followed by microscopic evaluation
- Lepromin test (intradermal reaction to heat-killed organisms)
- Other tests for diagnosis of leprosy
  - PCR test for DNA amplification of *M leprae* and *Mycobaterium lepromatosis*
  - Serology test for detection of phenolic glycolipid-I antibody

- Immunohistochemical markers for the detection of the bacillus
- Electrophysiological nerve tests[2,3,34]

Pathology

- Tuberculoid pattern
  - Well-formed granulomas with epithelioid cells, lymphocytes, and Langhans giant cells
  - Cutaneous nerves are edematous
  - Bacilli are usually scarce
- Lepromatous pattern
  - Lack of well-formed granulomas
  - Infiltrate of macrophages (Virchow cells) containing many bacilli (globi) and lipid drops
  - Cutaneous nerves with lamination of the perineurium
- Borderline pattern
  - Varying degrees of features of both lepromatous and tuberculoid patterns
- *M leprae* can be demonstrated by Ziehl-Neelsen or Fite-Faraco stains (**Fig. 12**)
- Globoid masses containing large groups of leprosy bacilli (globi) observed in
  - 100% of patients with lepromatous lesions
  - 75% of patients with borderline-type lesions
  - Rare patients with tuberculoid lesions[36,38]

THERAPEUTIC OPTIONS

- WHO-recommended multidrug therapy (adult regimen)
  - Multibacillary leprosy
    - Rifampicin 600 mg once a month, dapsone 100 mg daily, clofazimine 300 mg once a month, and 50 mg daily for 12 months
  - Paucibacillary leprosy

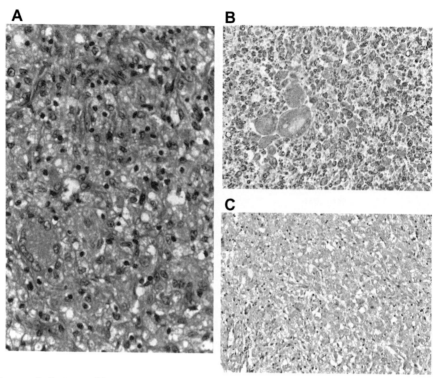

Fig. 12. Microscopic features of lepromatous leprosy characterized by (*A*) an infiltrate of macrophages and multinucleated giant cells, which were (*B*) positive for CD68, containing (*C*) many bacilli revealed by Ziehl-Neelsen staining (Hematoxylin and eosin, *A*, 400×; Immunoperoxidase, *B*, 100×; Ziehl-Neelsen, *C*, 100×).

- Rifampicin 600 mg once a month, dapsone 100 mg daily, clofazimine 300 mg once a month, and 50 mg daily for 6 months
  - Corticosteroids are the primary recommended treatment of leprosy reactions[34,39]

REFERENCES

1. Valour F, Senechal A, Dupieux C, et al. Actinomycosis: etiology, clinical features, diagnosis, treatment, and management. Infect Drug Resist 2014;7:183–97. https://doi.org/10.2147/IDR.S39601.
2. Neville BW, Damm DD, Allen CM, et al. Oral and Maxillofacial Pathology. 4th ed. Elsevier; 2016.
3. Farah CS, Balasubramaniam R, McCullough MJ. Non-odontogenic bacterial infections. *Contemporary Oral Medicine* Springer Nature; 2019. p. 873–928.
4. Karanfilian KM, Valentin MN, Kapila R, et al. Cervicofacial actinomycosis. Int J Dermatol 2020;59(10):1185–90. https://doi.org/10.1111/ijd.14833.
5. Lo Muzio L, Favia G, Lacaita M, et al. The contribution of histopathological examination to the diagnosis of cervico-facial actinomycosis: a retrospective analysis of 68 cases. Eur J Clin Microbiol Infect Dis 2014;33(11):1915–8. https://doi.org/10.1007/s10096-014-2165-0.
6. Moghimi M, Salentijn E, Debets-Ossenkop Y, et al. Treatment of cervicofacial actinomycosis: a report of 19 cases and review of literature. Med Oral Patol Oral Cir Bucal 2013;18(4):e627–32. https://doi.org/10.4317/medoral.19124.
7. Global tuberculosis report 2021. World Health Organization; 2021.
8. Prevention CfDCa. Trends in tuberculosis 2020. CDC. Available at: https://www.cdc.gov/tb/publications/factsheets/statistics/tbtrends.htm. Accessed 26 July 2022.
9. Salazar-Austin N, Dowdy DW, Chaisson RE, et al. Seventy Years of Tuberculosis Prevention: Efficacy, Effectiveness, Toxicity, Durability, and Duration. Am J Epidemiol 2019;188(12):2078–85. https://doi.org/10.1093/aje/kwz172.
10. Churchyard G, Kim P, Shah NS, et al. What We Know About Tuberculosis Transmission: An Overview. J Infect Dis 2017;216(suppl_6):S629–35. https://doi.org/10.1093/infdis/jix362.
11. Yepes JF, Sullivan J, Pinto A. Tuberculosis: medical management update. Oral Surg Oral Med Oral Pathol Oral Radiol Endod 2004;98(3):267–73. https://doi.org/10.1016/j.tripleo.2004.05.012.
12. Little JW, Falace DA, Miller CS, et al. Dental management of the medically compromised patient. Elsevier; 2013.
13. Centers for Disease Control and Prevention. Core curriculum on tuberculosis: what the clinician should know. CDC. Available at: https://www.cdc.gov/tb/

education/corecurr/pdf/CoreCurriculumTB-508.pdf. Accessed 26 July 2022.

14. Getahun H, Matteelli A, Chaisson RE, et al. Latent Mycobacterium tuberculosis infection. N Engl J Med May 28 2015;372(22):2127–35. https://doi.org/10.1056/NEJMra1405427.

15. Cadena AM, Fortune SM, Flynn JL. Heterogeneity in tuberculosis. Nat Rev Immunol 2017;17(11):691–702. https://doi.org/10.1038/nri.2017.69.

16. Wang WC, Chen JY, Chen YK, et al. Tuberculosis of the head and neck: a review of 20 cases. Oral Surg Oral Med Oral Pathol Oral Radiol Endod 2009;107(3):381–6. https://doi.org/10.1016/j.tripleo.2008.11.002.

17. Krawiecka E, Szponar E. Tuberculosis of the oral cavity: an uncommon but still a live issue. Postepy Dermatol Alergol 2015;32(4):302–6. https://doi.org/10.5114/pdia.2014.43284.

18. Kakisi OK, Kechagia AS, Kakisis IK, et al. Tuberculosis of the oral cavity: a systematic review. Eur J Oral Sci 2010;118(2):103–9. https://doi.org/10.1111/j.1600-0722.2010.00725.x.

19. de Farias Gabriel A, Kirschnick LB, So BB, et al. Oral and maxillofacial tuberculosis: A systematic review. Oral Dis 2022. https://doi.org/10.1111/odi.14290.

20. Papadogeorgakis N, Mylonas AI, Kolomvos N, et al. Tuberculosis in or near the major salivary glands: report of 3 cases. J Oral Maxillofac Surg 2006;64(4):696–700. https://doi.org/10.1016/j.joms.2005.11.035.

21. Sethi A, Sareen D, Sabherwal A, et al. Primary parotid tuberculosis: varied clinical presentations. Oral Dis Mar 2006;12(2):213–5. https://doi.org/10.1111/j.1601-0825.2005.01182.x.

22. Ficarra G, Carlos R. Syphilis: the renaissance of an old disease with oral implications. Head Neck Pathol 2009;3(3):195–206. https://doi.org/10.1007/s12105-009-0127-0.

23. Centers for Disease Control and Prevention. Sexually transmitted disease surveillance 2020. CDC. Available at: https://www.cdc.gov/std/statistics/2020/overview.htm#Syphilis. Accessed 30 July 2022.

24. Smith MH, Vargo RJ, Bilodeau EA, et al. Oral Manifestations of Syphilis: a Review of the Clinical and Histopathologic Characteristics of a Reemerging Entity with Report of 19 New Cases. Head Neck Pathol 2021;15(3):787–95. https://doi.org/10.1007/s12105-020-01283-4.

25. Leuci S, Martina S, Adamo D, et al. Oral Syphilis: a retrospective analysis of 12 cases and a review of the literature. Oral Dis 2013;19(8):738–46. https://doi.org/10.1111/odi.12058.

26. Kent ME, Romanelli F. Reexamining syphilis: an update on epidemiology, clinical manifestations, and management. Ann Pharmacother 2008;42(2):226–36. https://doi.org/10.1345/aph.1K086.

27. Centers for Disease Control and Prevention. Sexually transmitted infections treatment Guidelines. CDC. Available at: https://www.cdc.gov/std/treatment-guidelines/p-and-s-syphilis.htm. Accessed 30 July 2022.

28. Centers for Disease Control and Prevention. Group A Streptococcal (GAS) Disease. Available at: https://www.cdc.gov/groupastrep/diseases-hcp/scarlet-fever.html. Accessed 30 July 2022.

29. Castro MCR, Ramos ESM. The rash with mucosal ulceration. Clin Dermatol 2020;38(1):35–41. https://doi.org/10.1016/j.clindermatol.2019.10.019.

30. Workowski KA, Bachmann LH, Chan PA, et al. Sexually Transmitted Infections Treatment Guidelines, 2021. MMWR Recomm Rep 2021;70(4):1–187. https://doi.org/10.15585/mmwr.rr7004a1.

31. Kirkcaldy RD, Weston E, Segurado AC, et al. Epidemiology of gonorrhoea: a global perspective. Sex Health 2019;16(5):401–11. https://doi.org/10.1071/SH19061.

32. Tran J, Ong JJ, Bradshaw CS, et al. Kissing, fellatio, and analingus as risk factors for oropharyngeal gonorrhoea in men who have sex with men: A cross-sectional study. EClinicalMedicine 2022;51:101557. https://doi.org/10.1016/j.eclinm.2022.101557.

33. Unemo M, Shafer WM. Antimicrobial resistance in Neisseria gonorrhoeae in the 21st century: past, evolution, and future. Clin Microbiol Rev 2014;27(3):587–613. https://doi.org/10.1128/CMR.00010-14.

34. Chaves LL, Patriota Y, Soares-Sobrinho JL, et al. Drug Delivery Systems on Leprosy Therapy: Moving Towards Eradication? Pharmaceutics 2020;(12):12. https://doi.org/10.3390/pharmaceutics12121202.

35. Ghosh S, Gadda RB, Vengal M, et al. Oro-facial aspects of leprosy: report of two cases with literature review. Med Oral Patol Oral Cir Bucal 2010;15(3):e459–62. https://doi.org/10.4317/medoral.15.e459.

36. Motta AC, Komesu MC, Silva CH, et al. Leprosy-specific oral lesions: a report of three cases. Med Oral Patol Oral Cir Bucal 2008;13(8):E479–82.

37. Vohra P, Rahman MSU, Subhada B, et al. Oral manifestation in leprosy: A cross-sectional study of 100 cases with literature review. J Fam Med Prim Care 2019;8(11):3689–94. https://doi.org/10.4103/jfmpc.jfmpc_766_19.

38. Rodrigues GA, Qualio NP, de Macedo LD, et al. The oral cavity in leprosy: what clinicians need to know. Oral Dis 2017;23(6):749–56. https://doi.org/10.1111/odi.12582.

39. World Health Organization. Guidelines for the diagnosis, treatment and prevention of leprosy. Available at: https://www.who.int/publications/i/item/9789290226383. Accessed 24 July 2022.

Herpesvirus-Related Lesions of the Oral Mucosa

Shokoufeh Shahrabi-Farahani, DDS, MS, DMSc*, Sarah Aguirre, DDS, MS

KEYWORDS

- Humans • Herpesviridae • DNA viruses • Immunocompromised host • Coinfection
- Communicable diseases

KEY POINTS

- Herpesvirus-related lesions should be considered in the differential diagnosis of oral ulcerations.
- The appearance of clusters of coalescing ulcers due to rupture of vesicles following prodromal symptoms is the classic presentation of herpes simplex virus infection.
- Although herpes infection is a self-limiting process, systemic antiviral medication administered within the first 72 hours of symptom onset reduces the severity and duration of clinical disease.
- Midline termination of vesicles/ulcers is highly suggestive of herpes zoster.
- Immunocompromised patients are at higher risk for herpesvirus infections and may benefit from antiviral prophylaxis.

INTRODUCTION

At least 100 species of herpesviruses have been described in the nature but only 8 of those can infect humans, known as human herpesviruses (HHVs). Herpesviruses are double-stranded DNA-containing viruses in which the genome is surrounded by a capsid, tegument, and envelop. All are characterized by the establishment of latency in sensory nerves.[1]

There are 3 subfamilies of herpesviruses: The α-herpesviruses are those with a short (hours) replicative cycle and that are able to destroy host cells promptly and replicate in a wide variety of host tissues. This subfamily consists of herpes simplex virus (HSV) types 1 and 2 and varicella-zoster virus (VZV). The second subfamily is β-herpesviruses. Cytomegalovirus (CMV), and human herpes viruses 6 and 7 belong to this family. These viruses are characterized by a long (days) replicative cycle and restricted host range. Υ-herpesviruses are the third class and include Epstein-Barr virus (EBV) and human herpesvirus 8 (HHV-8). These have the most limited host range and can cause infections in certain targeted cells.[1]

HHVs and their associated lesions/diseases are summarized in **Table 1**.[1–6]

HERPES SIMPLEX VIRUS INFECTION
Introduction

The group of herpes simplex viruses (HSV) includes HSV-1 and HSV-2. Although both types of viruses have similar structure and share 50% to 70% of their genetic profiles, they are distinguished based on antigenic properties.[1] Both HSV-1 and HSV-2 infections can affect mucocutaneous surfaces, the central nervous system (CNS), and visceral organs.[7] Both viruses can cause similar primary or recurrent/recrudescent infections in the oral or genital regions. HSV-1 primarily affects mucosal sites including oral mucosa and skin above the waist, whereas HSV-2 predominantly affects mucosal sites including urogenital and skin below the waist[8] The highest incidence

Department of Diagnostic Sciences, University of Tennessee Health Science Center, College of Dentistry, 875 Union Avenue, Memphis, TN 38103, USA
* Corresponding author.
E-mail address: sfarahan@uthsc.edu

Oral Maxillofacial Surg Clin N Am 35 (2023) 175–187
https://doi.org/10.1016/j.coms.2022.10.012

Table 1
Herpesvirus-related conditions

Herpes Virus Type	Oral Lesion	Other Manifestation
HHV-1 Herpes simplex virus (HSV)-1	• Primary herpetic gingivostomatitis • Recurrent herpes labialis • Recurrent/recrudescent herpes stomatitis	• Herpetic whitlow • Herpes gladiatorum • Herpes encephalitis • Ocular herpes • Eczema herpeticum • Herpes esophagitis
HHV-2 Herpes simplex virus (HSV)-2	May cause oral lesions identical to those of HSV-1	• Lesions on skin and mucosal sites below the waist (genital) • Herpetic whitlow • Neonatal infection
HHV-3 VZV	• Possible oral ulcers caused by primary infection as chickenpox • Possible unilateral lesions due to the shingles (recrudescent infection) along the distribution of the branches of trigeminal nerve	• Skin lesions in primary infection (chickenpox) • Shingles due to activation of the latent virus • Acute neuritis • Postherpetic neuralgia • Severe complications in immuno-compromised patients
HHV-4 EBV	• IM • OHL (tongue) • EBV-related chronic oral ulcers in immunocompromised or immuno-senescent patients	• Nasopharyngeal carcinoma • Burkitt lymphoma • Hodgkin lymphoma • Angio-immunoblastic T-cell lymphoma • T/NK cell lymphoma • Nasal T/NK cell lymphoma • Plasmablastic lymphoma • EBV-associated chronic ulcers (EBV-associated, B-cell lymphoproliferative disorder)
HHV-5 CMV	Deep oral ulcers	• IM-like syndrome • Congenital cytomegalic inclusion disease • Severe complications in immuno-compromised patients
HHV-6 and HHV-7	No reported oral lesions	Roseola (exanthema subitum, sixth disease) with rejection of transplanted kidneys
HHV-8	KS	• AIDS-related lymphomas of organ cavities • Castleman disease

Data from Refs.[1–6]

of HSV-1 infection occurs after 6 months of age due to the loss of maternal anti-HSV antibodies and peak incidence is between 2 and 3 years of age. HSV-1 seroprevalence is 70% to 90% in populations of low socioeconomic status versus 40% to 60% in those with a higher socioeconomic status. HSV-2 infection typically presents after the onset of sexual activity and seroprevalence increases with age. Geographic, racial, socioeconomic, and ethnic characteristics among the general population may affect the seropositivity for HSV-2.[1,9–12] Recent data suggests declining seroprevalence of both HSV-1 and HSV-2 in the United States (US) and elsewhere.[7]

Pathogenesis

Oral HSV-1 infection is a common worldwide disease.[12] The main route of transmission is through saliva or direct contact with an active lesion.[8] Breaks in the epithelial barrier caused by mechanical or chemical injury can result in infection of a susceptible host. In up to 90% of cases, primary HSV infection is subclinical or causes a mild pharyngitis mimicking other upper respiratory viral or bacterial infections.[1,8] On entry of the virus into the oral mucosa or skin, and an incubation period of 4 to 6 days, HSV initially replicates in the epithelial cells and causes intraepithelial vesicle formation through the process of acantholysis. Then the virus migrates through sensory nerve axons to a dorsal root ganglion such as the trigeminal sensory ganglion where it remains latent indefinitely.

Primary Herpetic Stomatitis

Primary HSV infection may be symptomatic in subset of the patients, mostly observed in children and young adults and manifest as gingivostomatitis, which is preceded by prodromal symptoms including fever, sore throat, malaise, headache, gastrointestinal symptoms, and cervical lymphadenopathy. Within 1 to 2 days after the onset of the prodrome, the patient initially develops gingivitis and erythematous gingiva, followed by the formation of numerous vesicles within 2 to 3 days. The vesicles quickly rupture, giving rise to painful ulcers covered by yellowish white pseudomembrane. Both keratinized and nonkeratinized mucosa can be affected. Viral shedding occurs in the saliva during active disease. Gingiva, tongue, labial mucosa, palate, and the pharynx are the most common sites of involvement. The ulcers heal spontaneously in 7 to 10 days (**Figs. 1** and **2**).[1,2,6,8]

Clinically, primary herpetic gingivostomatitis may mimic other viral vesiculoulcerative processes such as hand-foot-and-mouth disease or herpangina, which are primarily seen in children, or certain autoimmune/immune-mediated vesiculoulcerative disorders. Patient age and the presence of prodromal symptoms can help to exclude autoimmune vesiculoulcerative processes.[2]

Secondary Herpetic Stomatitis

Reactivation of HSV-1 causes secondary (recurrent/recrudescent) lesions. During reactivation of the virus, retrograde axonal spread of the virus back to the skin or oral mucosa takes place along peripheral sensory nerves. Replication of the virus within the epithelium leads to vesicle development. Triggering factors for reactivation include exposure to cold, heat, sunlight, tissue trauma (such as trauma induced by dental procedures or local anesthetic injection), fever, stress, medications, or immunosuppression.[1,2,6,8,11,12] Along with other upper-respiratory infections, recent data have shown coronavirus disease-2019 may have a role in the reactivation of HSV.[13]

The most common form of recurrent HSV-1 infection is herpes labialis (colloquially referred to as a cold sore or fever blister), which is characterized by clusters of vesicles appearing on the mucocutaneous junction of the lip, perioral, or perinasal skin that rupture to a crusted or

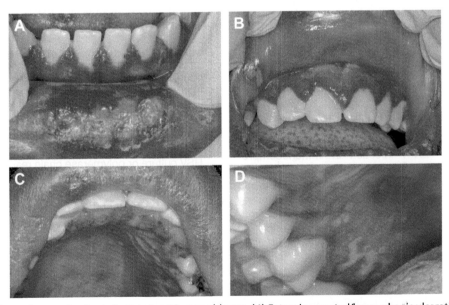

Fig. 1. Primary herpes simplex infection in a 23-year-old man. (*A*) Extensive crusted/hemorrhagic ulceration of the lower lip mucosa and generalized gingivitis of the mandibular gingiva. (*B*) Generalized maxillary gingivitis and ulcers on the right upper lip mucosa. (*C*) Multiple ulcers on the upper lip and generalized erosion with coalescing ulcers of the palatal gingiva/palate. (*D*) Right palatal gingivitis and multiple, coalescing ulcers caused by ruptured vesicles.

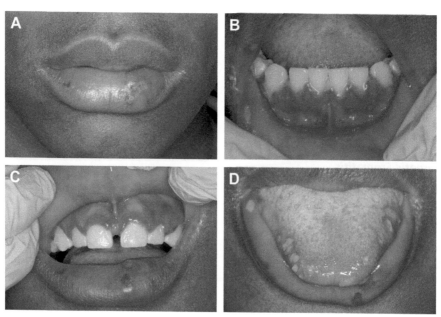

Fig. 2. Primary herpes simplex infection in a 19-year-old woman. (*A*) Crusted ulcerations on the left lower lip vermilion. (*B*) Ulcers on right upper and lower lip and generalized mandibular gingivitis with erosion/ulceration. (*C*) Generalized maxillary gingivitis and erosion with lower lip ulcers. (*D*) Multiple ulcers along the lateral borders of the tongue and lower lip.

hemorrhagic surface. Before the development of the vesicles, patients usually experience a prodromal burning/tingling sensation with an erythematous background (**Fig. 3**A).[1,2,6,8,12]

Intraoral recurrent HSV infection initially manifest as discrete solitary vesicles or multiple clustered vesicles. Typically, following rupture of the vesicles, coalescing ulcers form larger areas of ulceration with serpentine borders (**Fig. 3**B, C). Lesions in recurrent HSV infection usually last 7 to 10 days.[8]

Distinguishing features of primary and secondary HSV infections are shown in **Table 2**.

Herpes Simplex Virus and Immunocompromised Patients

Recurrent HSV-1 infection in immunocompromised patients may seem atypical as enlarging deep ulcers and can affect both keratinized and nonkeratinized mucosal sites, whereas in immunocompetent individuals, only the keratinized mucosa is involved.[8,11,12] The prevalence of recurrent oral HSV has been reported as 18% to 95% in organ transplant recipients.[14] Although the use of immunosuppressive medications has been shown to have an association with an increased risk of reactivation of HSV, using antiviral prophylactic regimens demonstrates efficacy in the prevention and reduction of recurrent HSV episodes in immunocompromised patients.[7] However, close monitoring is recommended to prevent

adverse treatment effects. Interestingly, the use of mTOR (mammalian target of rapamycin) inhibitors may results in decreased HSV reactivation.[7]

Differential Diagnosis

Recurrent lesions may be misdiagnosed as recurrent aphthous ulcers, traumatic ulcers, or chemotherapy-associated ulcers.

Diagnosis and Laboratory Confirmation

Diagnosis of HSV infection is primarily made by clinical presentation; however, adjunctive diagnostic tests may be required for atypical presentations. These may include viral culture, cytologic evaluation, histopathologic studies, direct fluorescent assay, serologic tests, and PCR.[11]

HSV culture or polymerase chain reaction (PCR) studies are recommended for atypical or persistent oral ulcers in immunocompromised patients, regardless of whether there are preceding prodromal symptoms or herpes labialis present. Biopsy may be indicated to rule out other infectious causes such as CMV or deep fungal infection. Coinfection of HSV and CMV has been reported in immunosuppressed patients.[8,12]

Complications

Recurrent herpetic infection may be associated with complications such as erythema multiforme, herpetic pneumonia, and herpetic esophagitis. In

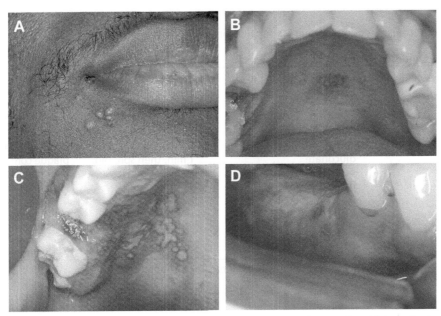

Fig. 3. Recurrent herpes simplex. (*A*) Herpes labialis in a 24-year-old man. Clusters of multiple coalescing ruptured and unruptured vesicles in the right commissural area and perioral skin. (*B*) Multiple coalescing ulcers on the hard palate in a 51-year-old woman. (*C*) Clusters of multiple coalescing ulcers in the right palatal gingiva/palate showing serpentine borders in a 22-year-old man. (*D*) Cluster of few, discrete ulcers in the mandibular gingiva/alveolar ridge mucosa in a 58-year-old man. (*Courtesy of* [*A*] Caroline Bissonnette, DDS, MS, Quebec, CA; [*C*] Masoud Hatami, DDS, MS, Kermanshah, IR.)

immunocompromised patients, it is possible for reactivation of HSV in a retrograde fashion from the ganglion to the CNS, leading to meningoencephalitis. There is also potential for dissemination and induction of a generalized infection.[1,8]

Treatment and Prognosis

Most HSV infections are self-limiting, requiring only symptomatic and supportive treatment. Antiviral treatment can reduce the severity of symptoms and accelerate the healing process. Antiviral medications may be effective if taken within 24 to 48 hours of lesion onset. Treatment regimens are shown in **Table 3**.[15–17]

VARICELLA-ZOSTER VIRUS

VZV (HHV-3) can cause 2 distinct disease presentations. Primary infection manifests as varicella (chickenpox). VZV then establishes latency in dorsal root/cranial nerve ganglia and may recur, typically decades later, as herpes zoster (HZ; shingles).[8]

Varicella (Chickenpox)

Varicella is highly contagious and easily spread through respiratory droplets or direct contact with vesicular fluid from active skin lesions.[8] Once a ubiquitous childhood infection with high

Table 2
Distinguishing features of primary and recurrent HSV infection

Features	Primary HSV	Recurrent HSV
Location	Both attached and unattached tissue	Attached, bone-bound tissue
Distribution	Widespread, diffuse	Localized, clustered
Number of lesions	Numerous	Fewer
Pain	Acute	Rarely
Treatment	Systemic antivirals	*Intraoral:* treatment usually unnecessary *Extraoral:* systemic antivirals

Table 3
Treatment recommendations for herpes simplex virus infection

Category/Condition	Medication	Dispense	Sig	Notes
Palliative/Primary or recurrent HSV	Lidocaine 2% viscous	100 mL	Swish with 15 mL for 1 min, then spit. As needed, no more than every 3 h to relieve pain	
	Chlorhexidine gluconate oral rinse 0.12%	473 mL	Swish with 15 mL for 1 min, then spit, bid. Use until oral lesions are no longer symptomatic	In addition to aiding in plaque control while pain may interfere with mechanical plaque removal, chlorhexidine displays synergistic antiviral effects with acyclovir
Systemic antiviral/Primary HSV[a]	Valacyclovir 1 g or	14–20 tablets	Take 1 tablet bid for 7–10 d	Valacyclovir is generally preferred over acyclovir due to the less frequent dosing schedule
	Acyclovir 400 mg	21–30 tablets	Take 1 tablet tid for 7–10 d	
Systemic antiviral/recurrent HSV[a]	Valacyclovir 500 mg or	16 tablets**	Take 4 tablets at the first sign of disease and then 4 tablets 12 h later	**The dispensed number of tablets for recurrent herpes episodes is double the amount needed for 1 episode. The additional tablets are available to take at the first sign of a subsequent episode for maximum effectiveness of the medication
	Acyclovir 400 mg	30 tablets**	Take 1 capsule tid for 5 d, beginning at the earliest sign of disease	
Topical antiviral	Docosanol cream 10%	2-g tube	Rub gently onto the affected area of the lip 5 times per day until the sore has healed	Initiate when symptoms first occur
Prophylaxis (acute)[a]	Valacyclovir 500 mg	6 tablets	Take 1 tablet bid (The day before the dental procedure, the day of the dental procedure, and the day after)	
Prophylaxis (chronic)[a]	Valacyclovir 500 mg	30 tablets	Take 1 tablet once daily	Reassess need periodically

[a] Systemic antiviral therapy should be used with caution in patients with renal impairment, the elderly, and/or those receiving nephrotoxic agents; dosing adjustments may be necessary.
Data from Refs.[15–17]

disease burden, the implementation of varicella vaccination has resulted in marked reductions in incidence, hospitalization, and mortality rate.[18–20] Recommendations in the US include the routine administration of a 2-dose varicella vaccine for children.[21]

In areas with high vaccine uptake, cases of varicella most often represent breakthrough infections due to infection with wild-type VZV.[8] Severity, extent, and duration of the clinical presentation are significantly decreased.[20]

Clinical Presentation

In unvaccinated individuals, the incubation period after exposure ranges from14 to 21 days.[20] A generalized, pruritic rash, often accompanied by mild fever and malaise is often the first sign of disease in children. The rash begins on the face/trunk, spreading to the extremities with rapid progression during 24 hours from macules to papules to vesicular lesions that crust over.[20] Among unvaccinated individuals, oral and perioral involvement is common.[22] The lip vermilion and palate are most often affected, followed by the buccal mucosa, labial mucosa, and tongue.[22] Lesions present as painless 2 to 4 mm vesicles that quickly rupture to shallow, flat-based yellowish-white to brown coalescing ulcers with erythematous halos.[22]

Diagnosis

Routine cases of varicella in unvaccinated children are diagnosed by clinical presentation. Breakthrough/atypical presentations may require laboratory confirmation.[8] Cytologic changes identical to those observed in HSV infection may be demonstrated in the epithelial cells of active lesions, although the most definitive method for diagnosis is PCR.[8]

Treatment and Prognosis

Antiviral therapy is not routinely offered to vaccinated individuals with mild breakthrough infections or unvaccinated children with uncomplicated varicella; however, it may be indicated for children at higher risk for complications, adults, or the immunocompromised.[23]

Zoster (Shingles)

VZV may reactivate, causing a vesicular rash known as HZ.[8] Unlike the multiple recurrences of HSV, a single recurrence for VZV is routine.[8] The most significant risk factors for HZ are diminished cell-mediate immunity with increasing age and immunocompromise.[8,24]

Clinical Presentation

HZ characteristically occurs in a unilateral distribution and can affect any dermatome but most often occurs on the trunk and the face.[24] The clinical course of HZ may be subdivided into 3 phases: prodrome, acute, and chronic. Pain, pruritis, dysesthesia, or paresthesia along the affected dermatome signal the prodromal period as the virus travels down the nerve to the epithelium.[2,24] The acute phase begins 2 to 4 days later with the development of red maculopapular lesions of the skin of the affected dermatome. The papules evolve into vesicles that rupture and crust over in 7 to 10 days with a complete resolution of the rash and accompanying pain in 2 to 6 weeks.[24] The chronic phase of HZ is characterized by postherpetic neuralgia (PHN): lingering pain for at least 3 months following the acute presentation.[8] Although most individuals do not progress to the chronic phase, the risk for PHN increases with age.[25]

Oral findings of zoster (**Fig. 4**) are secondary to involvement of either the maxillary or mandibular branch of the trigeminal nerve.[2] The prodromal period can be diagnostically challenging because it may present as facial pain, tooth pain, or mucosal tingling.[8] The affected mucosa will develop multiple vesicles with surrounding erythema, which quickly rupture to form shallow, yellowish-white membrane-covered ulcers.[25] Rarely reported dental complications include devitalization of teeth, internal root resorption, tooth exfoliation, and osteonecrosis.[25] Tooth exfoliation and osteonecrosis may occur from 2 to 12 weeks after onset of acute disease.[25]

Herpes zoster ophthalmicus refers to VZV involvement of the ophthalmic division of the trigeminal nerve. Involvement of the tip, side, or root of the nose (Hutchinson sign) is a strong indicator for severe ocular complications.[8] Reactivation of VZV from the geniculate ganglion may lead to unilateral peripheral facial paralysis accompanied by vesicles on the ipsilateral ear or oral cavity—a rare presentation termed Ramsay Hunt syndrome.[2,8]

Diagnosis

Diagnosis of zoster is routinely made based on the clinical presentation and history. HSV is considered in the differential diagnosis; however, midline termination of VZV lesions easily differentiates the 2.[2] In cases where zoster-like pain presents in the absence of rash (zoster sine herpete), PCR is essential for diagnosis.[2,8]

Treatment and Prognosis

Treatment of HZ is aimed at reducing the severity and duration of pain, shortening the duration of active lesions, preventing new lesion formation,

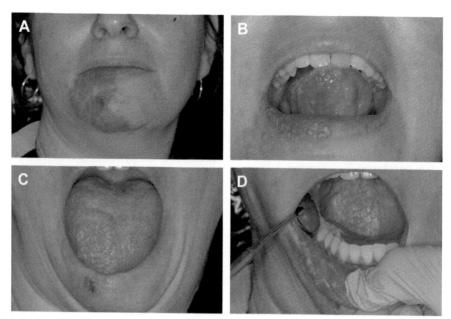

Fig. 4. HZ infection. (*A*) Unilateral multiple vesicles/ulcers with a background of erythema on the skin of right face and chin. (*B*) Unilateral ulcers/vesicles on the right lower lip vermilion, perioral skin, and right ventral tongue. (*C*) Unilateral ulcers on the right dorsal tongue, ending at the midline. (*D*) Right lower lip mucosa and dorsal tongue lesions.

and preventing PHN.[26] Therapy is most effective when initiated within 72 hours of rash onset with either acyclovir, valacyclovir, or brivudine.[26] Intravenous antivirals may be indicated in patients at risk for severe complications or immunocompromised individuals.[26] A combination of therapies, including gabapentin, tricyclic antidepressants, opioids, topical capsaicin, and topical lidocaine, may be used to manage PHN.[2,26] Management of dental complications may include endodontic therapy, tooth extraction, and conservative debridement of necrotic bone, in addition to antiviral therapy.[25] The 2-dose Shingrix recombinant zoster vaccine is recommended to adults aged 50 years or older and demonstrates substantial decreases in HZ disease burden, including incidence of PHN.[27]

EPSTEIN-BARR VIRUS
Introduction and Pathogenesis

EVB is a ϒ-herpesvirus responsible for several clinical entities.[1,10] EBV preferentially infects B lymphocytes and may be transmitted by intimate contact and saliva and respiratory secretions. More than 95% of adults are seropositive and chronically infected.[2]

Clinical Features of Epstein-Barr Virus Infection

During primary infection, EBV infects and replicates within the oropharyngeal epithelium and B lymphocytes.[2] Most infections of infants and children are symptomatic; however, infections in adolescents and adults results in symptomatic infectious mononucleosis (IM) after an incubation period of up to 8 weeks.[2] The clinical findings of IM consist of fever, malaise, myalgia, pharyngitis, palatal petechias, cervical lymphadenopathy, splenomegaly, and atypical lymphocytosis.[1,8]

Diagnosis

Diagnosis is confirmed by heterophile antibodies or type-specific antibodies against nuclear antigens and viral capsid antigens of EBV.[1]

Complications

Common complications of IM include myocarditis, hepatitis, hemolytic or aplastic anemia, thrombocytopenia, splenic rupture, and encephalitis.[2,28]

Treatment

The disease typically is mild and self-limiting and managed through supportive treatment but in cases with complications in immunocompetent patients, therapy may consist of a combination of antiviral and corticosteroids.[2]

EBV and Oral Mucosa: Pathogenesis, Clinical/ Histopathologic Features, and Treatment

EBV has been implicated in several epithelial and nonepithelial lesions and benign or malignant processes in the oral cavity.[4] The role of EBV has been established in oral hairy leukoplakia (OHL), undifferentiated nasopharyngeal carcinoma, and some lymphoproliferative disorders such as Burkitt lymphoma, EBV-positive large B-cell lymphoma, and T-cell/natural killer cell lymphoma, all of which may occur in oral mucosa or jaws.[4,8] EBV entry into epithelial cells is due to interactions of glycoproteins present in lipid envelop of the virus with host cells receptors such as neuropilin 1 (NRP1). NRP1 is expressed in nasopharyngeal epithelial cells and may promote EBV infection of these cells by coordinating receptor tyrosine kinase and macropinocytic events.[29] Although EBV mainly establishes latency in B lymphocytes, PCR studies have confirmed the presence of EBV latent infection in normal epithelium, gingivitis, epithelial dysplasia, and oral squamous cell carcinoma (SCC).[30–32] These findings suggest that the oral cavity is an environment that favors EBV infection.[4] Varied expression from 15% to 70% for latent EBV genes in oral SCC has been reported but the role of EBV in carcinogenesis has remained unclear.[30,31] During latency, different genes of EBV such as EBV-encoded small RNA (EBER) and latent membrane protein 1 (LMP-1) are expressed. These genes have role in oncogenesis. LMP-1 is critical for EBV-mediated B-cell transformation and is a major EBV-encoded oncogene.[4]

Aging, drug use, and organ transplantation result in EBV reactivation in the setting of decreased immunity.[4]

Oral Hairy Leukoplakia

OHL was first described in HIV-positive men.[33] Although OHL still highly indicates HIV seropositivity, it is also considered as an early indicator of EBV-associated posttransplant lymphoproliferative disorder (PTLD), and there are increasing cases of OHL in immunocompetent aging patients due to immunosenescence.[8,34,35] A recent report of OHL occurrence in 45 immunocompetent patients showed the role of aging or use of topical/systemic corticosteroids in the development of OHL, suggesting OHL evolution can result from localized, mild immunosuppression of the oral mucosa, possibly due to a decrease in the number of Langerhans cells.[34] Clinically, OHL seems as unilateral or bilateral white, corrugated plaques on the lateral or ventral tongue (**Fig. 5**). It may resemble frictional keratosis, lichen planus, cinnamon-induced hypersensitivity, or leukoplakia.[8,34] Histopathologically, OHL is characterized by corrugated hyperparakeratosis, epithelial hyperplasia, and nuclear beading observed in the superficial epithelial cells due to margination of

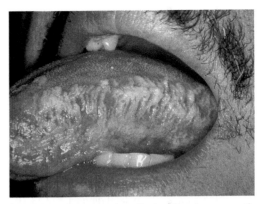

Fig. 5. OHL. Corrugated vertical white plaques on the left lateroventral tongue. (*Courtesy of* Sook-Bin Woo, DDS, MS, Boston, MA.)

chromatin, indicating of EBV replication.[34] Treatment is not necessary for this disease.[8]

Epstein-Barr Virus-Associated Lymphoproliferative Disorders

EBV-associated lymphoproliferative disorders (EBV-LPDs) occur in the setting of immunosuppression and decline in T cell-mediated immune surveillance, resulting in the expansion and transformation of an EBV-infected B cell reservoir.[4] EBV accounts for 90% of cases of PTLDs.[10] EBV-LPDs clinically manifest as masses involving various visceral organs, or ulcerative lesions on the skin or oral mucosa, termed EBV-positive mucocutaneous ulcer (EBVMCU).[3,10] Cases of EBVMCU have shown an association with immunosuppression induced by medications such as azathioprine, methotrexate, tumor necrosis factor-α antagonists, or cyclosporine-A, or aging.[3,4] EBV-associated oral ulcers clinically manifest as solitary or multiple, deep, sharply demarcated ulcers, mostly affecting the gingiva, tongue, lip, buccal mucosa, palate, and oropharynx (**Fig. 6**).[3,36] Histopathologically, these lesions are characterized by the presence of atypical B-cell blasts with Hodgkin/Reed-Sternberg morphology with strong positivity for CD30 and EBER positivity.[3] EBV-LPDs demonstrate indolent behavior and a self-limiting clinical course. Reducing immunosuppression and withdrawal of the medication may result in complete remission of the process. Treatment with immunomodulating agents such as rituximab, IL-6, and interferon-α has also been reported. Antiviral medication may decrease the risk of EBV-induced PTLD.[3,37,38]

CYTOMEGALOVIRUS INFECTION
Systemic Manifestations

CMV causes 3 distinct diseases. Congenital cytomegalic inclusion disease affects approximately

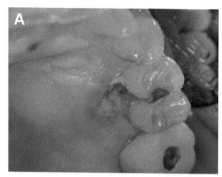
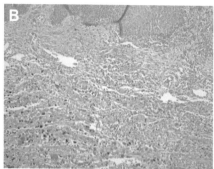

Fig. 6. EBV-related chronic oral ulcer in a 92-year-old man with history of taking methotrexate. (*A*) A deep, well-demarcated ulcer on the palatal gingiva, #12-13. (*B*) In situ hybridization (ISH) demonstrating EBV-infected cells. (ISH, ×100 total magnification). (*Courtesy of* [*A*] Lee Hinson, DDS, MAGD, Little Rock, AR.)

1% of newborns and may cause severe symptoms in 10% of the infected children.[1] Symptoms include petechial/purpuric skin rash (due to thrombocytopenia), hepatosplenomegaly, retinitis, and involvement of the CNS.[1] The second disease caused by CMV is a type of mononucleosis syndrome, which can cause symptomatic primary infection in 10% of infected teenagers and adults.[1] In contrast to EBV-related IM, patients with this disease lack specific antibodies to the viral antigens of EBV. The clinical symptoms are similar to those caused by EBV but cervical lymphadenopathy or hepatitis is rarely present. The third manifestation of CMV infection is seen in the setting of immunosuppression caused by either HIV infection or after bone marrow or solid organ transplantation. This type of infection may be serious and life-threatening and can involve several organs and tissues such as the lungs, oral mucosa, and salivary glands.[1,2,6,39] The relationship between hyposalivation/xerostomia and the presence of CMV in saliva of HIV-infected patients has been reported, possibly due to salivary gland infection and dysfunction caused by the virus.[40,41]

The genomes of the 2 herpesviruses of EBV and CMV have been demonstrated in some severe forms of periodontitis including HIV-associated periodontitis and necrotizing ulcerative granuloma, which indicates the possible role of these viruses in the pathogenesis and progression of periodontal disease, possibly through the production of cytokines involved in bone loss and interference with collagen formation and the healing process.[42]

Oral Manifestations

CMV-related oral lesions may be chronic, painful, enlarging, punched out, and penetrating ulcers, without surrounding edema. These usually involve palate, gingiva, tongue, and floor of the mouth but any mucosal site can be affected.[2,6,8,39]

Pathogenesis

During the primary infection, CMV tends to infect a variety of cells and tissues such as epithelial cells, endothelial cells, T-lymphocytes, CNS, and glandular tissues, including the salivary glands and the kidneys, and establishes latency in the monocytes/macrophages.[43] Persistent infection with CMV has been reported in salivary glands, breast tissue, kidneys, endocervix tissue, seminal vesicles, and peripheral blood leukocytes, which results in chronic viral excretion by the involved tissue. Therefore, transmission may occur via mother to child, infected breast milk, saliva, cervical secretion, urine, and blood transfusion.[1]

Diagnosis and Histopathologic Features

Diagnosis of CMV disease is made by histopathologic studies of suspected lesions, viral culture, antigen detection, and PCR. Histopathologically, CMV infection is characterized by the presence of multinucleated giant cells (endothelial cells or salivary duct epithelium) exhibiting both intranuclear (Cowdry inclusions) and intracytoplasmic inclusion bodies. These cells may be described as "owl-eye" cells.[6,8,39]

Treatment

Ganciclovir has been shown to be effective for the treatment of CMV infection in immunocompromised patients.[1,2,6]

KAPOSI SARCOMA-ASSOCIATED VIRUS (HHV-8)

HHV-8 is a ϒ-herpesvirus responsible for Kaposi sarcoma (KS) as well as primary effusion lymphoma and some forms of Castleman disease.[10] The seroprevalence of HHV-8 is variable and is

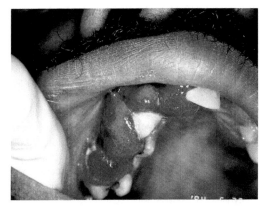

Fig. 7. KS in a patient with AIDS. Lobulated red/purple nodular lesion of the right maxillary gingiva. (*Courtesy of* Sook-Bin Woo, DDS, MS, Boston, MA.)

highest among homosexual men. Sexual activity and saliva are considered as the primary routes of transmission of this virus.[10] HHV-8 may also be transmitted by organ transplantation, and KS is the most common malignancy seen in renal transplant recipients.[6,10] KS is a malignancy of vascular origin and classically presents as multiple red-purple plaques or nodules, usually affecting the skin of the lower extremities in men aged older than 60 years but in AIDS-associated KS, the gingiva, palate, and tongue are the common sites of involvement.[8] The initial stages of the disease seem as single or multifocal macules that then progresses to plaques, and finally grow to nodules, which may mimic pyogenic granuloma (**Fig. 7**).[2,8] Clinical progression is positively associated with the viral load.[44] Oral KS may be the first manifestation of an undiagnosed HIV infection.[2]

SUMMARY

Six members of the HHV family, including HSV-1, HSV-2, VZV, EBV, CMV, and HHV-8 can cause a variety of oral lesions, ranging from common to rare presentations, affecting epithelial or nonepithelial tissues. HHV causes primary infection when the patient is initially exposed to the virus, then establishes latency in a variety of cells. Through reactivation, triggered by factors such as trauma and immunosuppression, recurrent lesions may develop. HHV may have a significant role in the etiology of oral mucosal infectious diseases in immunocompromised patients. Although some HHV-induced oral lesions are self-limiting, those that occur in immunocompromised patients may be life-threatening and lead to complications that may necessitate antiviral treatment or antiviral prophylaxis.

CLINICS CARE POINTS

- Systemic antiviral treatment initiated during the prodromal period of recurrent HSV may prevent the development of vesicles/ulcers, therefore additional medication should be prescribed for the patient to have on-hand to take at the first sign of a recurrent episode.

- If dental care is a known trigger for reactivation of HSV, a prophylactic antiviral regimen should be initiated the day before the dental appointment.

- HSV is transmissible until all lesions have crusted over—elective dental care should be postponed if active lesions are present.

- Stark midline termination of vesicles or ulcers is pathognomonic for HZ.

- Lesional involvement of HZ of the tip, side, or root of the nose is a strong indicator for ocular complications and necessitates referral to an ophthalmologist.

- Oral EBV-LPDs may mimic other benign and malignant lesions, clinically or histopathologically. Therefore, accurate diagnosis of such lesions is crucial to avoid unnecessary patient management. The diagnosis requires a comprehensive correlation between patient's medical/medication history, clinical findings, and histopathologic features including immunohistochemical and in situ hybridization studies.

FUNDING SOURCES

No funding sources.

DISCLOSURE

The authors have nothing to disclose.

REFERENCES

1. Whitley RJ. Medical Microbiology. Fourth ed. Galveston: University of Texas Medical Branch; 1996.
2. Balasubramaniam R, Kuperstein AS, Stoopler ET. Update on oral herpes virus infections. Dent Clin North Am 2014;58(2):265–80.
3. Dojcinov SD, Venkataraman G, Raffeld M, et al. EBV positive mucocutaneous ulcer–a study of 26 cases associated with various sources of immunosuppression. Am J Surg Pathol 2010;34(3):405–17.
4. Kikuchi K, Inoue H, Miyazaki Y, et al. Epstein-Barr virus (EBV)-associated epithelial and non-epithelial lesions of the oral cavity. Jpn Dent Sci Rev 2017;53(3):95–109.

5. Stojanov IJ, Woo SB. Human papillomavirus and Epstein-Barr virus associated conditions of the oral mucosa. Semin Diagn Pathol 2015;32(1): 3–11.

6. Stoopler ET. Oral herpetic infections (HSV 1-8). Dent Clin North Am 2005;49(1):15–29, vii.

7. Lee DH, Zuckerman RA. Herpes simplex virus infections in solid organ transplantation: Guidelines from the American Society of Transplantation Infectious Diseases Community of Practice. Clin Transpl 2019;33(9):e13526.

8. Neville BWDD, Allen CM, Chi AC. Oral and Maxillofacial Pathology. Fourth ed. Canada: Elsevier; 2016.

9. Crimi S, Fiorillo L, Bianchi A, et al. Herpes Virus, Oral Clinical Signs and QoL: Systematic Review of Recent Data. Viruses 2019;11(5).

10. Shiley K, Blumberg E. Herpes viruses in transplant recipients: HSV, VZV, human herpes viruses, and EBV. Infect Dis Clin North Am 2010;24(2):373–93.

11. Stoopler ET, Sollecito TP. Oral mucosal diseases: evaluation and management. Med Clin North Am 2014;98(6):1323–52.

12. Woo SB, Lee SF. Oral recrudescent herpes simplex virus infection. Oral Surg Oral Med Oral Pathol Oral Radiol Endod 1997;83(2):239–43.

13. Shanshal M, Ahmed HS. COVID-19 and Herpes Simplex Virus Infection: A Cross-Sectional Study. Cureus 2021;13(9):e18022.

14. Schubert MM, Peterson DE, Flournoy N, et al. Oral and pharyngeal herpes simplex virus infection after allogeneic bone marrow transplantation: analysis of factors associated with infection. Oral Surg Oral Med Oral Pathol 1990;70(3):286–93.

15. Gilbert SC. Suppressive therapy versus episodic therapy with oral valacyclovir for recurrent herpes labialis: efficacy and tolerability in an open-label, crossover study. J Drugs Dermatol 2007;6(4): 400–5.

16. Park NH, Park JB, Min BM, et al. Combined synergistic antiherpetic effect of acyclovir and chlorhexidine in vitro. Oral Surg Oral Med Oral Pathol 1991; 71(2):193–6.

17. Wald AJC, Hirsch MS, Mitty J. Treatment and prevention of herpes simplex virus type 1 in immunocompetent adolescents and adults. 2022. Available at: https://www.uptodate.com/contents/treatment-and-prevention-of-herpes-simplex-virus-type-1-in-immunocompetent-adolescents-and-adults.

18. Davis MM, Patel MS, Gebremariam A. Decline in varicella-related hospitalizations and expenditures for children and adults after introduction of varicella vaccine in the United States. Pediatrics 2004;114(3): 786–92.

19. Leung J, Marin M. Update on trends in varicella mortality during the varicella vaccine era-United States, 1990-2016. Hum Vaccin Immunother 2018;14(10): 2460–3.

20. Lopez A HT, Marin M. Varicella. In: Epidemiology and prevention of vaccine-Preventable diseases. 14th ed.2021:329-347.

21. Marin M, Güris D, Chaves SS, et al. Prevention of varicella: recommendations of the Advisory Committee on Immunization Practices (ACIP). MMWR Recomm Rep 2007;56(Rr-4):1–40.

22. Kolokotronis A, Louloudiadis K, Fotiou G, et al. Oral manifestations of infections of infections due to varicella zoster virus in otherwise healthy children. J Clin Pediatr Dent 2001;25(2):107–12.

23. American Academy of Pediatrics. Varicella-Zoster Infections. In: Kimberlin DW, Barnett ED, Lynfield R, Sawyer MH, editors. *Book: 2021-2024 Report of the Committee on Infectious Diseases.* 32nd ed. Itasca, IL: American Academy of Pediatrics; 2021. p. 831–42.

24. Leung JHT, Dooling K. Herpes Zoster. In: Epidemiology and prevention of vaccine-Preventable diseases. Centers for Disease Control and Prevention, Public Health Foundation; 2021. p. 348–58.

25. Kaur R, Rani P, Malhotra D, et al. A rare case report and appraisal of the literature on spontaneous tooth exfoliation associated with trigeminal herpes zoster. Oral Maxillofac Surg 2016;20(3):331–6.

26. Patil A, Goldust M, Wollina U. Herpes zoster: A Review of Clinical Manifestations and Management. Viruses 2022;14(2).

27. Dooling KL, Guo A, Patel M, et al. Recommendations of the Advisory Committee on Immunization Practices for Use of Herpes Zoster Vaccines. MMWR Morb Mortal Wkly Rep 2018;67(3):103–8.

28. Maakaroun NR, Moanna A, Jacob JT, et al. Viral infections associated with haemophagocytic syndrome. Rev Med Virol 2010;20(2):93–105.

29. Wang HB, Zhang H, Zhang JP, et al. Neuropilin 1 is an entry factor that promotes EBV infection of nasopharyngeal epithelial cells. Nat Commun 2015;6: 6240.

30. Gonzalez-Moles MA, Gutierrez J, Rodriguez MJ, et al. Epstein-Barr virus latent membrane protein-1 (LMP-1) expression in oral squamous cell carcinoma. Laryngoscope 2002;112(3):482–7.

31. Higa M, Kinjo T, Kamiyama K, et al. Epstein-Barr virus (EBV)-related oral squamous cell carcinoma in Okinawa, a subtropical island, in southern Japan-simultaneously infected with human papillomavirus (HPV). Oral Oncol 2003;39(4):405–14.

32. Slots J, Saygun I, Sabeti M, et al. Epstein-Barr virus in oral diseases. J Periodontal Res 2006;41(4): 235–44.

33. Greenspan D, Greenspan JS, Conant M, et al. Oral "hairy" leucoplakia in male homosexuals: evidence of association with both papillomavirus and a herpes-group virus. Lancet 1984;2(8407):831–4.

34. Almazyad A, Alabdulaaly L, Noonan V, et al. Oral hairy leukoplakia: a series of 45 cases in

immunocompetent patients. Oral Surg Oral Med Oral Pathol Oral Radiol 2021;132(2):210–6.

35. Casiglia J, Woo SB. Oral hairy leukoplakia as an early indicator of Epstein-Barr virus-associated post-transplant lymphoproliferative disorder. J Oral Maxillofac Surg 2002;60(8):948–50.

36. Kunmongkolwut S, Amornkarnjanawat C, Phattarataratip E. Multifocal Oral Epstein-Barr Virus-Positive Mucocutaneous Ulcers Associated with Dual Methotrexate and Leflunomide Therapy: A Case Report. Eur J Dent 2022;16(3):703–9.

37. Karras A, Thervet E, Legendre C. Hemophagocytic syndrome in renal transplant recipients: report of 17 cases and review of literature. Transplantation 2004;77(2):238–43.

38. Lee ES, Locker J, Nalesnik M, et al. The association of Epstein-Barr virus with smooth-muscle tumors occurring after organ transplantation. N Engl J Med 1995;332(1):19–25.

39. Fitzpatrick SG, Cohen DM, Clark AN. Ulcerated Lesions of the Oral Mucosa: Clinical and Histologic Review. Head Neck Pathol 2019;13(1):91–102.

40. Greenberg MS, Dubin G, Stewart JC, et al. Relationship of oral disease to the presence of cytomegalovirus DNA in the saliva of AIDS patients. Oral Surg Oral Med Oral Pathol Oral Radiol Endod 1995; 79(2):175–9.

41. Greenberg MS, Glick M, Nghiem L, et al. Relationship of cytomegalovirus to salivary gland dysfunction in HIV-infected patients. Oral Surg Oral Med Oral Pathol Oral Radiol Endod 1997; 83(3):334–9.

42. Slots J, Contreras A. Herpesviruses: a unifying causative factor in periodontitis? Oral Microbiol Immunol 2000;15(5):277–80.

43. Plachter B, Sinzger C, Jahn G. Cell types involved in replication and distribution of human cytomegalovirus. Adv Virus Res 1996;46:195–261.

44. Feller L, Lemmer J. Insights into pathogenic events of HIV-associated Kaposi sarcoma and immune reconstitution syndrome related Kaposi sarcoma. Infect Agent Cancer 2008;3:1.

Lichenoid Lesions of the Oral Mucosa

Nadim M. Islam, DDS, BDS*, Saja A. Alramadhan, BDS

KEYWORDS

- Chronic ulcerative stomatitis • Oral lichen planus • Lichenoid drug eruptions
- Graft-versus-host disease

KEY POINTS

- Understand the clinical presentation of lichenoid lesions of the oral mucosa.
- Develop insight into the demographics of these lesions and correlate the clinical presentation with the histopathology.
- Identify possible lichenoid lesions and be familiar with management options.
- Understand the clinical variability and discriminate lichenoid lesions from vesiculo-bullous diseases.

CHRONIC ULCERATIVE STOMATITIS

Chronic ulcerative stomatitis (CUS) is a rare immune-mediated mucocutaneous disease involving the mucosal surfaces and rarely, the skin. It was first described in 1989 by Beutner and colleagues[1] and later reported by Jaremko and colleagues[2] in 1990 as a unique entity characterized by the presence of oral erosive or ulcerative lesions with an excellent clinical response to hydroxychloroquine. CUS and erosive oral lichen planus (ELP) have overlapping clinical and histologic features. The only method to distinguish cases of ELP from CUS is direct immunofluorescence (DIF) or indirect IF (IIF) testing. It is important to discriminate CUS from ELP and autoimmune bullous diseases as CUS is highly refractory to corticosteroid therapy or routine management.[3,4]

The prevalence of CUS may be more common than is realized due to misdiagnosis. Biopsies may be submitted for routine light microscopy alone, and the DIF studies essential for diagnosis of CUS may not be requested. A total of 80 CUS cases have been reported in the worldwide English language literature.[1–16]

CLINICAL FEATURES

CUS has an array of clinical presentations that are similar to both oral lichen planus (OLP; **Fig. 1**) and autoimmune bullous diseases.[3,4,12,16] In the oral cavity, CUS manifests clinically as nonhealing ulcerative or erosive lesions with or without desquamative gingivitis (**Fig. 2**).[3,12,16] The 91.5% of cases reported in the English language literature involve white women, with an average age of 60.6 years (range 22–84 years). The condition is common in the fifth and sixth decades of life. Almost all areas in the oral cavity may be involved with the buccal mucosa, gingiva, and the tongue being the most commonly affected areas (**Figs. 3** and **4**). Other locations include the palate, lingual mucosa, lower lip, and cheek (**Fig. 5**).[3,4,12,16] At least 22.5% of cases reported in the English language literature had extraoral involvement.[4] The condition generally presents as progressive painful, erythematous gingival lesions, with large, tender erosions, ulcerations, and vesicle formation as well as hypertrophic areas especially on the tongue dorsum mimicking hypertrophic lichen planus (LP) (**Figs. 6–8**). The ulcers are surrounded by zones of

Department of Oral and Maxillofacial Diagnostic Sciences, University of Florida College of Dentistry, 1395 Center Drive, Gainesville, FL 32610, USA
* Corresponding author. UF College of Dentistry, 1395 Center Drive, Gainesville, FL 32610.
E-mail address: mnislam@ufl.edu

Oral Maxillofacial Surg Clin N Am 35 (2023) 189–202
https://doi.org/10.1016/j.coms.2022.10.005
1042-3699/23/© 2022 Elsevier Inc. All rights reserved.

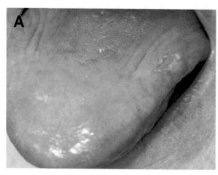
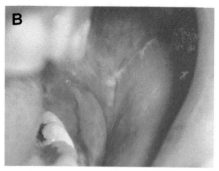

Fig. 1. (*A*) CUS involving the left lateral tongue as an ulcer with a yellowish center surrounded by a diffuse whitish border. (*B*) Same patient with lesions exhibiting diffuse white striae involving the left buccal mucosa resembling lichen planus.

erythema and streaky keratosis that resemble OLP, although classic striae formation is not evident. The ulcers heal without scarring with periods of alternating severity and migration around the oral mucosa.[3–5,12,16] These clinical features overlap with ELP and autoimmune diseases, including benign mucous membrane pemphigoid (MMP), pemphigus vulgaris (PV), and systemic lupus erythematosus (LE).

Patients usually suffer from varying degrees of discomfort including nervousness, fatigue, and inability to consume sweet, salty foods, hot, or cold drinks as well as a rare few with dry mouth. Some patients suffer from weight loss and sleeplessness. They may also experience malaise, depression, apathy, and a feeling of helplessness.[3–5,9,12,16]

DIAGNOSIS AND HISTOPATHOLOGIC FEATURES

CUS cases under routine microscopy exhibit histopathologic overlap with LP. Ulcerated specimens

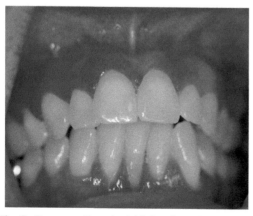

Fig. 2. Desquamative gingivitis involving both maxillary and mandibular facial gingiva.

exhibiting atrophic epithelium with few saw-toothed rete ridges and an eosinophilic coagulum along the basement membrane zone are not uncommon (**Fig. 9**). Numerous eosinophilic Civatte bodies (necrotic keratinocytes) are also seen within the epithelium. Significant interface stomatitis (leukocytic exocytosis) with partial destruction of the basal cell layer may be seen. As these features may be similar to the findings of several other epithelial separation diseases, DIF testing remains the mainstay of diagnosis.[3,4,12,16]

Immunofluorescence Studies

The final diagnosis of CUS is based on DIF testing that shows a speckled, finely granular pattern of Immunoglobulin G (IgG) staining in basal and parabasal cell nuclei of keratinocytes (**Figs. 10** and **11**). DIF studies of lesional and perilesional oral mucosal specimens are consistently positive on DIF for IgG in the stratified epithelium in a specific, ANA pattern (see **Figs. 1, 10, 11**; Fig. **12**). This signal is confined to the basal and parabasal cells (lower third) of the spinous layers. DIF staining of IgG was observed in 80% of the patients and 67.5% showed a nuclear stratified epithelium-specific ANA pattern.[3,4,12,16]

All oral erosive and/or ulcerative lesions, nonresponsive, to standard therapies, and exhibiting histopathologic features suggestive of LP, should be subjected to DIF testing.

IIF is also positive for these stratified epithelium-specific ANA. An ezyme-linked immunosorbent assay (ELISA) test has been developed and possibly will make screening for this condition much more cost-effective if commercially available.[3–6,8,15,17,18]

TREATMENT AND PROGNOSIS

The unique feature of CUS is the response to hydroxychloroquine.[3,4,12,16,19] The lesions

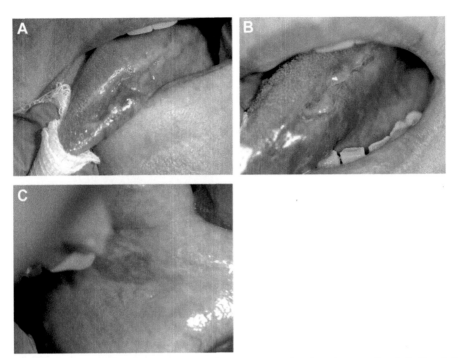

Fig. 3. (*A, B*) Deep, linear ulceration with whitish and erythematous borders that may be clinically misdiagnosed as erosive lichen planus. (*C*) Ulceration surrounded by plaque-like borders (lichenoid pattern) on the left buccal mucosa.

commonly heal and regress uneventfully. Hydroxychloroquine limits the disease progression/persistence and patients generally remain asymptomatic. Antimalarial drugs, though effective initially, cannot be continued over a prolonged period due to gastrointestinal and/or ocular side effects. Also, hydroxychloroquine should be used cautiously to prevent side effects such as retinopathy, toxic psychosis, neuromyopathy, agranulocytosis, and aplastic anemia. Periodic ophthalmologic and hematologic evaluation is prudent and if adverse reactions noted discontinuation of therapy is recommended.[3,12,16,19] The neuromuscular and hematologic complications are reversible, but retinal complications are irreversible and mandates close follow-up for patients on hydroxychloroquine therapy. A dosage of 200 mg/day helps improve the condition in most of the cases and a sizable number of oral lesions are completely cured.[3,4,12,16,19] A variety of topical steroids such as fluocinonide, betamethasone, clobetasol, dexamethasone elixir, and dapsone have been used to treat CUS with some general improvement of symptoms. Dapsone, however, has severe gastrointestinal side effects so patients should be scheduled for clinical follow-up within 12 weeks.[3,12,16]

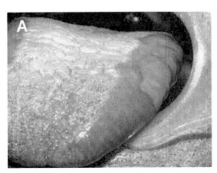
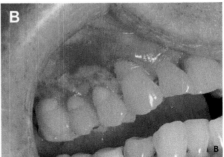

Fig. 4. (*A*) Large, shallow ulcers involving the lateral tongue. (*B*) Involvement of the gingiva showing exhibiting erosive, ulcerated areas that resemble periodontal disease.

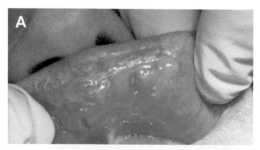

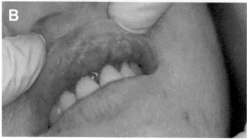

Fig. 5. (A, B) CUS involving lips; crusted lips with ulcerations that clinically might be misdiagnosed as erythema multiform or herpes simplex virus infection.

Clinicians and oral health care providers should remain sentient about the possibility of CUS, especially when dealing with recalcitrant and debilitating cases of oral ulcers, unresponsive to empirical therapy.

ORAL LICHEN PLANUS

LP is an autoimmune condition that affects the skin, hair, eyes, mucous membranes, and nails and was initially described in 1869 by British physician Wilson Erasmus.[20] The lesions of LP on the skin have a purplish raised flat almost plaque-like, papular appearance and are mostly pattern less. Oral lesions are termed OLP, and almost

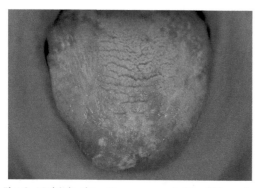

Fig. 6. Multiple ulcerations surrounded by diffuse plaque-like white lesions resembling hypertrophic lichen planus.

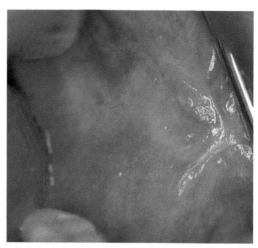

Fig. 7. Left buccal mucosa, ulcerations with lichenoid appearance.

53.6% of cutaneous LP patients may present with oral lesions.[20,21] Erosive OLP lesions appear as inflamed ulcerations with a white linear or lacy pattern. It may be seen in only one area but exhibits a tendency to migrate within the mouth or skin over time.[20–22] The lesions are seen to "wax" and "wane" and are characterized by periods of remission followed by flare-ups. The active periods are symptomatic in some cases. This presents a significant challenge for the patient to eat, drink, and function due to the constant pain.[20–23] OLP is more common in women over the age of 40 and in non-Asian countries.[21] It is a chronic T-cell-mediated disease of the oral mucosa. Increased numbers of mast cells with significant degranulation are a consistent finding in OLP.[20–23] Lichenoid lesions can be distinguished from true LP as they often have an identifiable causative agent. Among the several possible causative agents for lichenoid lesions, pharmaceuticals and dental materials are the most common. Resolution of the lesions with removal of the potential causative agent is conformational for lichenoid reaction. However, if lesions continue, a diagnosis of LP/OLP is rendered.[22,24,25]

CLINICAL FEATURES

LP affects predominantly middle-aged adult women (ratio, 3:2 over men) and is rare in children.[20,21] Cutaneous LP affects 1% of the population, whereas OLP has a prevalence between 0.1% and 2.2%. Cutaneous LP is characterized by as the 4 Ps: purple, pruritic, polygonal papules, that usually affect the flexor surfaces of the extremities. Like cutaneous LP, OLP presents as a

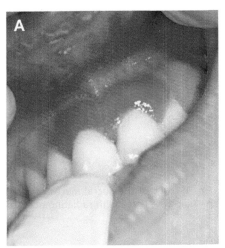
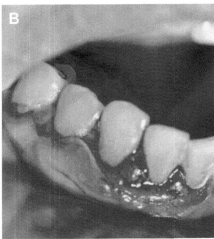

Fig. 8. (*A*) Localized gingival erythema. (*B*) Severe erosion presenting as desquamative gingivitis.

fine, lacelike network of white lines (Wickham striae) with adjacent erythematous zones (**Fig. 13**).[20–25]

OLP has two forms: reticular and erosive. Reticular LP is much more common, but the erosive form due to its symptomatic nature and hence referral bias predominates the literature.[20,21,26] The reticular form is usually asymptomatic and involves the posterior buccal mucosa bilaterally (**Fig 14**). Post-inflammatory melanin incontinence may be seen along with the reticular striae, especially with the chronic erosive form and among people of color.[20–23] Other oral mucosal surfaces affected include the lateral border of the tongue, the gingivae, the palate, and the vermilion border of

the lip (**Figs. 15–17**). OLP lesions of the tongue dorsum are unique and present as thick, white to greyish-white keratotic plaques and may cause atrophy of the tongue papillae (**Fig. 18**).[20–25]

Erosive lichen planus (ELP) is relatively uncommon but more significant due to its symptomatic nature. Clinically, these present as atrophic, erythematous areas bordered by fine white striae that is radiating with mostly central ulceration (**Fig. 19**). These lesions occasionally are limited to the gingiva and in the erosive form are termed desquamative gingivitis (**Fig. 20**).[26] ELP is most often associated with medications.[24–26] Unlike with vesiculo-bullous (VB)-diseases, biopsy for OLP should involve striae if possible and avoid

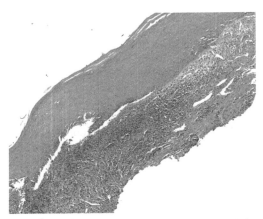

Fig. 9. Hematoxylin and eosin-stained section exhibiting atrophic epithelium, focal separation with lichenoid lymphocytic infiltrate, and thin parakeratosis (magnification X10).

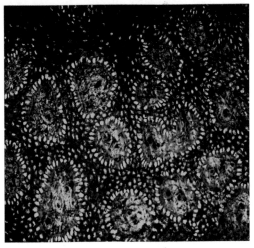

Fig. 10. SES-ANA pattern of IgG antibodies deposition in the basal epithelial cell nuclei, on a transversely sectioned specimen (magnification X40).

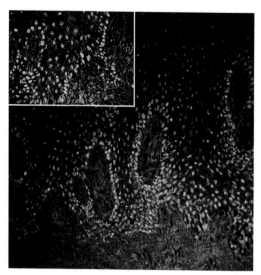

Fig. 11. Speckled pattern of IgG antibodies in the epithelium (magnification X20). Inset shows the speckled nuclear deposition of IgG antibodies in the basal and parabasal epithelial cells (magnification X40).

ulcerated areas. This is important to rule out other erosive entities such as MMP and PV that may present in a similar fashion.

DIAGNOSIS AND HISTOPATHOLOGIC FEATURES

The diagnosis of OLP is variable and usually based on the subtype. The reticular type is usually diagnosed based on the clinical findings alone. The

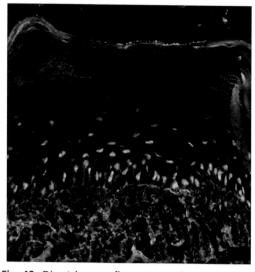

Fig. 12. Direct immunofluorescence showing deposition of IgG antibody in the basal and parabasal epithelial nuclei (magnification X20).

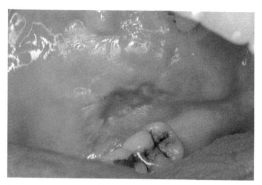

Fig. 13. OLP of the buccal mucosa exhibiting erosive and ulcerated area with radiating mild striations.

presentation of bilaterally appearing interlacing white striae of the posterior buccal mucosa is pathognomonic.[20–22] Lesions may be confounded by superimposed candidal infection that may alter the typical reticular pattern (Fig. 21).[22,26]

The more challenging diagnosis involves ELP, especially if based only on clinical features. In cases with radiating white striae along with red, erythematous mucosa and ulcerations, a strong presumptive clinical diagnosis of ELP may be rendered. This can be done at times without additional biopsy/histopathologic findings. In many instances, however, a biopsy, often with DIF studies, is warranted to rule out other overlapping entities such as LE or CUS.[3,20–23] Asymmetric or isolated erosive lichenoid lesions, particularly those of the soft palate, the lateral and ventral tongue, or the floor of the mouth, should always be biopsied to rule out premalignant changes or malignancy.[26,27] Several other conditions exist that may mimic an isolated lesion of LP, both clinically and histopathologically. These included lichenoid reaction to graft-versus-host disease (GVHD), LE, CUS, and oral mucosal cinnamon reaction.[21,24,25]

On H & E sections, the surface epithelium may be orthokeratotic and/or parakeratotic. The thickness of the spinous layer may vary and if present rete ridges may have a pointed or "saw-toothed" shape (Fig. 22A). Hydropic degeneration of the basal cell layer is a hallmark which is accompanied by an intense, bandlike infiltrate composed predominantly of T-lymphocytes located immediately subjacent to the epithelium (Fig. 22A).[20,22] Few to several necrotic keratinocytes called Civatte bodies are appreciated within the epithelium or the subjacent lamina propria.[20] A classic OLP biopsy seldom will exhibit epithelial dysplasia; however, lesions with superimposed candidal infection may appear erythematous and worrisome. When located in high-risk locations, this presentation

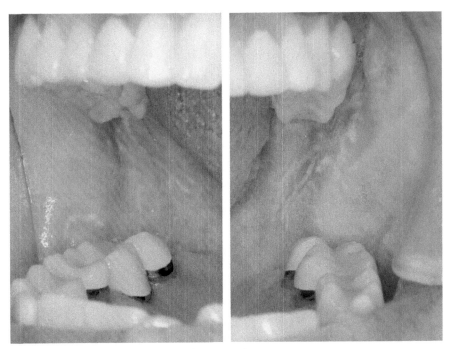

Fig. 14. Classic OLP with bilateral buccal mucosal presentation.

may be challenging and should be revisited following appropriate antifungal therapy.[20] It is sometimes confusing when dealing with dysplastic lesions as the host response to the dysplastic epithelium demonstrates a similar lichenoid infiltrate.[27,28] This may be challenging to pathologists and can cause significant misinterpretation. The overlapping histologic and even clinical features of dysplasia and LP may fuel the controversy related to the potential malignant transformation of LP. Direct immunofluorescent studies will exhibit deposition of a shaggy bandlike fibrinogen presence at the basement membrane zone (**Fig. 22**B).[20–26] This is true only if there is a good epithelial-connective tissue junction without any separation.[20–22]

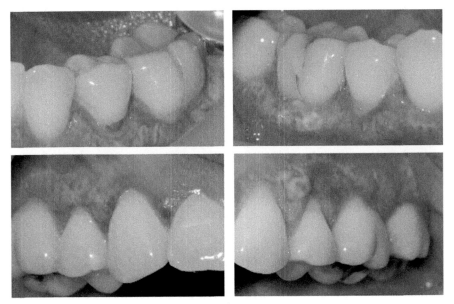

Fig. 15. Gingival presentation of OLP with leukoplakic features.

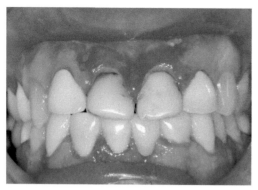

Fig. 16. ELP lesions presenting as desquamative gingivitis.

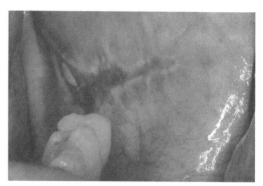

Fig. 19. Posterior buccal mucosal lesion with erosive and ulcerated area and prominent white radiating striations.

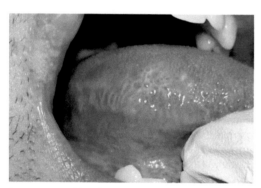

Fig. 17. Lateral border of the tongue exhibiting reticular lichen planus with classic white striations.

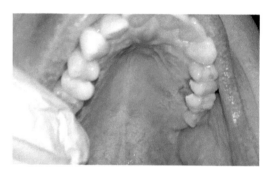

Fig. 20. Left palatal presentation of reticular lichen planus.

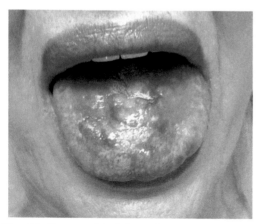

Fig. 18. Hypertrophic lichen planus of the dorsal tongue.

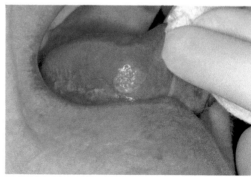

Fig. 21. Erosive lichen planus lesions of the right lateral border of tongue.

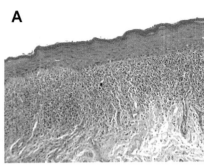

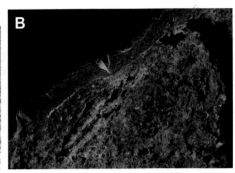

Fig. 22. (*A*) Hematoxylin and eosin-stained section of OLP with atrophic epithelium, bandlike lymphocytic infiltrate. (*B*) Direct immunofluorescence showing bandlike fibrinogen at the epithelial-connective tissue interface.

TREATMENT AND PROGNOSIS

For asymptomatic, symmetric reticular LP with no therapeutic intervention is required. If a superimposed candidal infection is suspect due to clinical symptom of burning and/or erythema, antifungal therapy is indicated. It is, however, recommended that reticular lichen planus (RLP) patients be followed up annually. ELP is usually symptomatic and as it is immunologically mediated, corticosteroids are the mainstay of therapy. ELP responds to systemic corticosteroids well, but this is not recommended except in severe cases. The favorite mode of treatment, therefore, is using stronger topical corticosteroids (eg, fluocinonide, betamethasone, or clobetasol gel). The protocol includes using a thin film applied to the area 2 to 4 times per day, especially on the most symptomatic area. This regimen often resolves the lesion(s) within 1 or 2 weeks. A tapered application method is the most judicious method.[20–26] It is important that patients are made aware that lesions might recur, and they may need to retreat the area. If lesions fail to heal or only partially respond search for an underlying causative medication is recommended. In addition, the potential of immunosuppressive therapy-related fungal infection remains strong, and hence, close monitoring is warranted.[20] If a long-term ELP patient suddenly worsens one of two things is the likely cause: candidal colonization or malignant transformation.[27,28] A combination therapy including corticosteroid ointments along with an adhesive methylcellulose base is cumbersome to use due to difficulty in application and therefore, not popular. Other not so widely used strategies include agents such as topical retinoids, tacrolimus, mycophenolate mofetil, or cyclosporine. These have been used for recalcitrant cases of ELP but with limited success.[21,22] Oral ELP patients should be evaluated every 3 to 6 months, especially, if the condition worsens, the lesions are asymmetric, and/or the clinical presentation/location of involvement appears unusual.[26–28] Treatment with both topical and systemic glucocorticosteroids is used for the most severe cases. While uncommon, localized steroid injections can be used in cases that do not respond to topical or systemic treatment.[20–26]

The potential for malignant transformation of OLP is not entirely clear. It is important to consider whether the lesions were true LP as leukoplakic

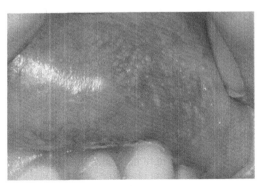

Fig. 23. Lichenoid lesion of the lip.

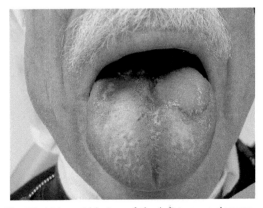

Fig. 24. Lichenoid lesion of the left tongue dorsum.

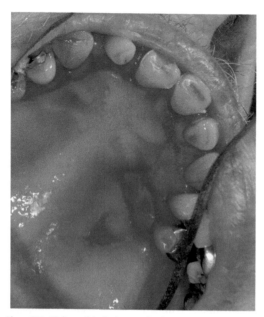

Fig. 25. Lichenoid lesion of the anterior palatal gingiva.

lesions that are truly dysplastic may present with a lichenoid inflammatory infiltrate and both microscopically and clinically mimic LP. It is worth mentioning that there is only at best a small 1% to 3% potential for malignant transformation and only the red erosive or atrophic lesions are known to transform.[20–22,27,28]

LICHENOID DRUG ERUPTIONS

Oral lichenoid drug eruption or drug-induced lichenoid lesions (OLDE) share some common clinical and histological presentations with oral LP.[22,25] Unlike classical LP, OLDE have a causative association with a drug(s) or medication(s), and although they may have striae or white lines, they are often asymmetric in distribution.[22,24,25,29–31] Health care professionals must

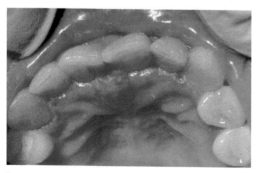

Fig. 26. Deep craterlike lichenoid ulceration of the left hard palate

recognize these differences, especially as OLDE treatment depends on identifying the trigger/causative agent rather than the standard topical steroid therapy for oral LP. Over 80% of patients with so-called erosive LP are taking drug(s) that is likely the cause of their lichenoid eruption.[29–31] OLDE usually have a predominant erosive component, and unlike classical reticular LP, it is invariably symptomatic. The lesions appear atrophic, erythematous with areas of central ulceration (**Figs. 23–26**) and are bordered by fine, white radiating striae (**Fig. 27**A–D).[29,30]

Lichenoid drug eruptions are difficult to diagnose because these reactions are complex and very different from the typical drug allergy and several drugs can cause this problem.[22,24,25,29–31] Furthermore, many patients are on multiple medications that can cause this reaction. However, several caveats may help reach a correct diagnosis. Unlike the typical drug allergies that develop almost immediately, OLDE take an average of 6 to 12 months to develop. Even more unusual, OLDE can develop after 10 years of receiving the same medication(s). In addition, OLDE lesions may ebb and flow (wax and wane), whereas patients continue taking their medication(s), which is most uncharacteristic for a drug allergy. Also, OLDE usually have an asymmetric eruption pattern and tend to occur commonly on the buccal mucosa, and lower lip, and rarely on the tongue and palate.[29–31]

In general, antihypertensive and non-steroidal anti inflammatory drugs (NSAID) are the most common causative agents. However, OLDE lesions are strictly dependent on many factors such as patients' susceptibility, age, gender, dosage, and the pharmacological action of a drug.[29,30]

DIAGNOSIS AND HISTOPATHOLOGIC FEATURES

OLDE diagnosis can be confirmed by withdrawal of the suspected medication(s), if medically feasible, and regression of the lesion.[29–31]

The histological features of OLDE are similar to that of oral LP, however, the inflammatory infiltrate is more diffuse and located deeper in the lamina propria. There is a tendency for perivascular inflammation with the infiltrate not limited to lymphocytes but mixed with plasma cells and occasionally eosinophils.[22,25,29,30]

TREATMENT AND PROGNOSIS

Withdrawal of the right causative agent may bring about the desired result within 2 to 8 weeks, but some patients may take up to 24 months to

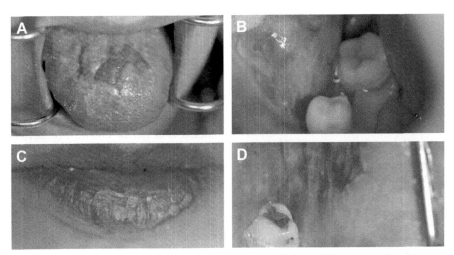

Fig. 27. (*A–D*) Lichenoid drug eruptions with erosive and ulcerated lesions of the tongue, buccal mucosa, and the lip.

become free of the lesions. Topical corticosteroids such as clobetasol propionate ointment along with good oral hygiene and the use of antiseptic mouth rinses may help relieve the symptoms.[29–31]

GRAFT-VERSUS-HOST DISEASE

GVHD is a complication triggered by the reactivity of donor-derived immune cells against allogeneic recipient tissues. The skin, liver, eyes, gastrointestinal tract, lungs, and joints are typically affected. GVHD mainly occurs following allogeneic bone marrow transplantation. However, GVHD may also occur following a blood transfusion, organ transplant, or face transplant. [32–36] Based on the clinical features and the timing of presentation, GVHD is classified into acute and chronic. Overlap syndrome is a phenomenon in which acute and chronic GVHDs occur simultaneously.[32] Acute GVHD is characterized by erythema, maculopapular rash of the skin, hepatitis, jaundice, and gastrointestinal tract symptoms, that is, nausea, vomiting, abdominal pain, diarrhea, and/or anorexia all within 100 days of transplant. One or more organs may be involved.[32–36] The chronic form is characterized by the involvement of a number of organs, including the oral cavity which may be the only affected location in chronic GVHD. The presentation may include lichenoid lesions, hyperkeratotic plaques, and inability to open the mouth due to sclerotic changes. The oral condition is usually mild, but moderate to severe erosive and ulcerated lesions may be seen. The diagnosis is based on clinical characteristics, though biopsy helps confirmation in some cases. Oral involvement in GVHD is nonspecific and may mimic other autoimmune diseases/lesions.[32–36]

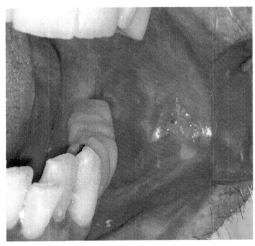

Fig. 28. Lesion of GVHD on the buccal mucosa.

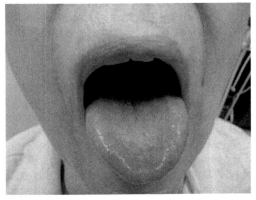

Fig. 29. Faint lesion of the tongue dorsum in a patient with GVHD. Notice the subtle depapillation.

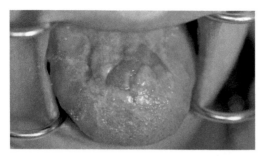

Fig. 30. Severely ulcerated, erosive, and erythematous lesion of the tongue dorsum on a GVHD patient.

CLINICAL FEATURES

Lesions may present as erythematous/erosive areas with ulcers and/or as white striae that resemble LP. The buccal mucosa, tongue, and lips are the most commonly affected oral sites (**Figs. 28–30**). Desquamative gingivitis may be also seen, with or without white reticulation. Oral lesions especially during acute GVHD may be painful. The presence of these often painful oral lesions may impair oral hygiene resulting in dental plaque-induced gingivitis and may increase oral erythema and ulcerations.[33–36]

DIAGNOSIS AND HISTOPATHOLOGIC FEATURES

GVHD is a clinicopathologic diagnosis based strongly on presentation and patients' medical history.[32] According to the National Institutes of Health (NIH) consensus paper, a biopsy for GVHD is done to rule out other conditions, such as dysplasia or cancer.[37] White plaque-like lesions were removed from the list of diagnostic criteria of oral acute GVHD in the 2014 NIH consensus paper so as to ensure that white dysplastic or malignant lesions are not misdiagnosed and presumed to be manifestations of GVHD.[38] The microscopic features of GVHD are nonspecific but often resemble LP. The superficial patchy bandlike inflammatory infiltrate is much milder than that seen in LP.[35]

TREATMENT AND PROGNOSIS

The most common therapeutic agents for GVHD are corticosteroids. Owing to the increased risk of fungal superinfection with steroid use, concomitant antifungal therapy is recommended. An important goal in treatment is an early detection of malignant changes, as patients with chronic oral GVHD are at high risk.[32–37] Biannual screening is recommended by the NIH.[37] Corticosteroids such as a budesonide 0.03%–0.06% mouthwash has been reported to be effective for oral lesions.

Dexamethasone 0.01% mouth rinse is a somewhat successful popular treatment alternative. The choice of therapy is based heavily on the extension and severity of lesions and most importantly the cost and patient preference and tolerance.[33–36]

For large-sized lesions, a solution is preferred, but if lesions are small or isolated the popular choice is a gel or cream. For severe cases, a high potency/systemic agent is the choice and occasionally a combination of systemic and topical agents may be warranted.[32–36,39] Intralesional triamcinolone injection is recommended for cases resistant to routine therapy.[39] Nonsteroidal agents and tacrolimus have been used for topical treatment of oral GVHD.[33–36]

CLINICS CARE POINTS

- If a lichenoid lesion fails to respond to topical steroids, consider chronic ulcerative stomatitis, which is a lichenoid lesion clinically and microscopically indistinguishable from erosive lichen planus diagnosed on DIF and requires treatment with hydroxychloroquine.

- Lichenoid lesions can be distinguished from true lichen planus as they often have an identifiable causative agent and pharmaceuticals (lichenoid drug eruption) and dental materials (amalgam) are the most common causative agents.

- Erosive lichen planus is most often associated with medications, and if lesions do not respond to topical steroid therapy clinicians should search for the causative drug.

- Unlike with VB-diseases, biopsy for OLP should involve striae if possible and avoid ulcerated areas.

- If a long-term ELP patient suddenly worsens one of two things is the likely cause: candidal colonization or malignant transformation.

- Patients with chronic oral GVHD are at high risk for malignancy and the oral cavity may be the only affected location.

DISCLOSURE

No financial support was provided for this work and the authors do not have conflicts of interest.

REFERENCES

1. Beutner EH, Chorzelski TP, Parodi A, et al. Ten cases of chronic ulcerative stomatitis with stratified

epithelium-specific antinuclear antibody. J Am Acad Dermatol 1991;24(5 Pt 1):781–2.

2. Jaremko WM, Beutner EH, Kumar V, et al. Chronic ulcerative stomatitis associated with a specific immunologic marker. J Am Acad Dermatol 1990; 22(2 Pt 1):215–20.

3. Chapter 14 chronic ulcerative stomatitis. In: Schmidt E, Islam MN, Alramadhan S, et al, editors. Diseases of the Oral Mucosa: Study Guide and Review E-textbook. Cham, Switzerland: Springer; 2021. p. 151–62.

4. Azzi L, Cerati M, Lombardo M, et al. Chronic ulcerative stomatitis: A comprehensive review and proposal for diagnostic criteria. Oral Dis 2019;25(6): 1465–91.

5. Alshagroud R, Neiders M, Kramer JM, et al. Clinicopathologic significance of in vivo antinuclear autoantibodies in oral mucosal biopsies. Oral Surg Oral Med Oral Pathol Oral Radiol 2017;124(5):475–82.

6. Cacciapuoti M, Di Marco E, Cozzani E, et al. The antibody to the 70-kd antigen in chronic ulcerative stomatitis and lichen planus. J Am Acad Dermatol 2004;50(3):486.

7. Carlson MW, Garlick JA, Solomon LW. Chronic ulcerative stomatitis: evidence of autoimmune pathogenesis. Oral Surg Oral Med Oral Pathol Oral Radiol Endod 2011;111(6):742–8.

8. Chorzelski TP. [Chronic ulcerative stomatitis (CUS): a new disease entity with specific immunological marker (SES-ANA)]. Przegl Dermatol 1990;77(4): 229–32.

9. Chorzelski TP, Olszewska M, Jarzabek-Chorzelska M, et al. Is chronic ulcerative stomatitis an entity? Clinical and immunological findings in 18 cases. Eur J Dermatol 1998;8(4):261–5.

10. Church LF, Schosser RH. Chronic ulcerative stomatitis associated with stratified epithelial specific antinuclear antibodies. A case report of a newly described disease entity. Oral Surg Oral Med Oral Pathol 1992;73(5):579–82.

11. Feller L, Khammissa RAG, Lemmer J. Is chronic ulcerative stomatitis a variant of lichen planus, or a distinct disease? J Oral Pathol Med 2017;46(10): 859–63.

12. Islam MN, Cohen DM, Ojha J, et al. Chronic ulcerative stomatitis: diagnostic and management challenges–four new cases and review of literature. Oral Surg Oral Med Oral Pathol Oral Radiol Endod 2007;104(2):194–203.

13. Lewis JE, Beutner EH, Rostami R, et al. Chronic ulcerative stomatitis with stratified epithelium-specific antinuclear antibodies. Int J Dermatol 1996;35(4): 272–5.

14. Parodi A, Cozzani E, Chorzelski TP, et al. A molecule of about 70 kd is the immunologic marker of chronic ulcerative stomatitis. J Am Acad Dermatol 1998;38(6 Pt 1):1005–6.

15. Parodi A, Cozzani E, Cacciapuoti M, et al. Chronic ulcerative stomatitis: antibodies reacting with the 70-kDa molecule react with epithelial nuclei. Br J Dermatol 2000;143(3):671–2.

16. Reddy R, Fitzpatrick SG, Bhattacharyya I, et al. Seventeen New Cases of Chronic Ulcerative Stomatitis with Literature Review. Head Neck Pathol 2019; 13(3):386–96.

17. Solomon LW, Neiders ME, Zwick MG, et al. Autoimmunity to deltaNp63alpha in chronic ulcerative stomatitis. J Dent Res 2007;86(9):826–31.

18. Solomon LW, Stark PC, Winter L, et al. ELISA test for p63 antibodies in chronic ulcerative stomatitis. Oral Dis 2010;16(2):151–5.

19. Stoopler ET, Kulkarni R, Alawi F, et al. Novel combination therapy of hydroxychloroquine and topical tacrolimus for chronic ulcerative stomatitis. Int J Dermatol 2021;60(4):e162–3.

20. Au J, Patel D, Campbell JH. Oral lichen planus. Oral Maxillofacial Surg Clin N Am 2013;25:93–100.

21. Andrea E, Reyes E, Al-Eryani K. Oral Lichen Planus: A review of clinical features, etiologies, and treatments. Dentistry Rev 2022;2(1):100007.

22. Al-Hashimi I, Schifter M, Lockhart PB, et al. Oral lichen planus and oral lichenoid lesions: diagnostic and therapeutic considerations. Oral Surg Oral Med Oral Pathol Oral Radiol Endod 2007; 103(Suppl):S25e1–25e12.

23. Belfiore P, Di Fede O, Cabibi D, et al. Prevalence of vulval lichen planus in a cohort of women with oral lichen planus: an interdisciplinary study. Br J Dermatol 2006;155:994–8.

24. Borghelli RF, Pettinari IL, Chuchurru JA, et al. Oral lichen planus in patients with diabetes: an epidemiologic study. Oral Surg Oral Med Oral Pathol 1993;75:498–500.

25. Giunta JL. Oral lichenoid reactions versus lichen planus. J Mass Dent Soc 2001;50(2):22–5.

26. Alrashdan MS, Cirillo N, McCullough M. Oral lichen planus: a literature review and update. Arch Dermatol Res 2016;308(8):539–51.

27. Accurso BT, Warner BM, Knobloch TJ, et al. Allelic imbalance in oral lichen planus and assessment of its classification as a premalignant condition. Oral Surg Oral Med Oral Pathol Oral Radiol Endod 2011;112:359–66.

28. Brzak BL, Mravak-Stipeti M, Canjuga I, et al. The frequency and malignant transformation rate of oral lichen planus and leukoplakia— a retrospective study. Coll Antropol 2012;36:773–7.

29. Halevy S, Shal A. Lichenoid drug eruptions. J Am Acad Dermatol 1993;29(2 Pt 1):249–55.

30. Woo V, Bonks J, Borukhova L, et al. Oral lichenoid drug eruption: a report of a pediatric case and review of the literature. Pediatr Dermatol 2009;26(4):458–64.

31. Fortuna G, Aria M, Schiavo JH. Drug-induced oral lichenoid reactions: a real clinical entity? A systematic review. Eur J Clin Pharmacol 2017;73:1523–37.

32. Kuten-Shorrer M, Woo SB, Treister NS. Oral graft-versus-host disease. Dent Clin North Am 2014;58: 351–68.

33. Treister NS, Cook EF Jr, Antin J, et al. Clinical evaluation of oral chronic graft-versus-host disease. Biol Blood Marrow Transplant 2008;14:110–5.

34. Imanguli MM, Pavletic SZ, Guadagnini JP, et al. Chronic graft versus host disease of oral mucosa: review of available therapies. Oral Surg Oral Med Oral Pathol Oral Radiol Endod 2006;101:175–83.

35. Margaix-Muñoz M, Bagán JV, Jiménez Y, et al. Graft-versus-host disease affecting oral cavity. A review. J Clin Exp Dent 2015;7(1):e138–45.

36. Elad S, Aljitawi O, Zadik Y. Oral Graft-Versus-Host Disease: A Pictorial Review and a Guide for Dental Practitioners. Int Dent J 2021;71(1):9–20.

37. Kitko CL, Pidala J, Schoemans HM, et al. National Institutes of Health Consensus Development Project on Criteria for Clinical Trials in Chronic Graft-versus-Host Disease: IIa. The 2020 Clinical Implementation and Early Diagnosis Working Group Report. Transpl Cell Ther 2021;27(7):545–57.

38. Jagasia MH, Greinix HT, Arora M, et al. National Institutes of Health Consensus Development Project on Criteria for Clinical Trials in Chronic Graft-versus-Host Disease: I. The 2014 Diagnosis and Staging Working Group report. Biol Blood Marrow Transplant 2015;21(3):389–401.e1.

39. Zadik Y. Pharmacotherapy of oral mucosal manifestations of chronic graft-versus-host disease: When? What? and How? Expert Opin Pharmacother 2020; 21(12):1389–92.

Vesiculobullous Lesions of the Oral Cavity

Saja A. Alramadhan, BDS*, Mohammed N. Islam, DDS, BDS

KEYWORDS

- Cicatricial pemphigoid • Pemphigus vulgaris • Epidermolysis bullosa acquisita
- Bullous pemphigoid • Desquamative gingivitis

KEY POINTS

- Recognize and distinguish the subtle clinical features of the vesiculobullous diseases.
- Develop a clear perception of the susceptible patient group or population.
- Understand the direct immunofluorescence diagnostic features attributed to each important vesiculobullous diseases.
- Become alert in recognizing the possibility of vesiculobullous diseases.
- Develop a global understanding of the etiologies and sharpen skills to manage vesiculobullous diseases.

INTRODUCTION

Vesiculobullous lesions involving the oral cavity may represent the oral manifestations of dermatologic diseases, particularly those that are immune-mediated. Several vesiculobullous conditions may affect the oral cavity, and they must be distinguished from other types of oral ulcerations as they may reflect systemic diseases and require special treatment. Desquamative gingivitis is a hallmark of the majority of vesiculobullous conditions especially benign mucous membrane pemphigoid (BMMP).[1–6] Histopathologic examination with direct immunofluorescence (DIF) studies is the gold standard for diagnosing autoimmune vesiculobullous conditions.[1–7] This article discusses the clinical features, pathogenesis, differential diagnosis, diagnostic features, histology, and immunofluorescence findings as well as management of vesiculobullous diseases. These diseases include pemphigus vulgaris (PV), BMMP, bullous pemphigoid (BP), and epidermolysis bullosa acquisita. They all have a significant impact on the quality of life and can lead to serious complications, depending on the extent of the disease. Therefore, early recognition is crucial to reduce disease-related morbidity and mortality and prevent life-threatening complications.

PEMPHIGUS VULGARIS

PV is an uncommon debilitating vesiculobullous disease characterized by flaccid bullae and erosions affecting the skin and/or mucous membrane. PV is one of the four-pemphigus variants, along with pemphigus vegetans, pemphigus erythematosus, and pemphigus foliaceus, with PV being the most common.[8,9] PV and pemphigus vegetans are the two variants that can affect oral mucosa, however, pemphigus vegetans is considered an extremely rare condition.[5,10] Patients of Mediterranean, South Asian, and Ashkenazi Jews heritages have higher rates of this condition. PV has an estimated prevalence of 30,000 cases in the United States and an incidence of 1 to 10 new cases per 1 million population.[8–11] The pathogenesis of PV is mediated by immunoglobulin G (IgG) autoantibodies directed against structural proteins of the desmosomes at cell–cell junctions. Patients who have developed autoantibodies targeting desmoglein 3 with or without desmoglein 1 will have cutaneous and mucosal disease, whereas patients

Department of Oral and Maxillofacial Diagnostic Sciences, University of Florida College of Dentistry, 1395 Center Drive, Room D8-06, Gainesville, FL 32610, USA
* Corresponding author.
E-mail address: salramadhan@dental.ufl.edu

Oral Maxillofacial Surg Clin N Am 35 (2023) 203–217
https://doi.org/10.1016/j.coms.2022.10.006
1042-3699/23/© 2022 Elsevier Inc. All rights reserved.

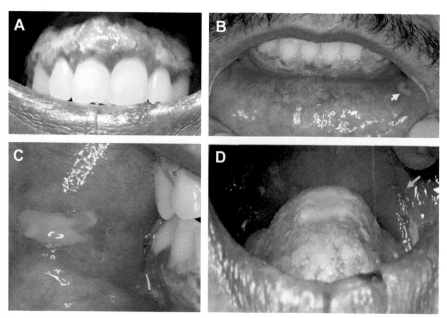

Fig. 1. Diffuse ulceration and mucosal sloughing are prominent on; (*A*) Facial maxillary gingiva and (*B*) facial mandibular gingiva with ulceration are noted on the left labial mucosa (*yellow arrow*). (*C*) Large ulceration of the right buccal mucosa. (*D*) Coated tongue and posterior palatal extension of ulcerations (*green arrow*).

with autoantibodies targeting only desmoglein 1 will only have cutaneous disease.[9]

PV is a potentially life-threatening disease with a mortality rate of 5% to 15%. Mortality is mainly due to treatment complications, skin infections, and pneumonia. Therefore, early diagnosis and treatment before extensive skin involvement is crucial.[8,11,12]

CLINICAL FEATURES

PV typically affects middle-aged patients, with an average age of 50 years, and equal gender distribution.[8,11,12] Rare cases have been reported in childhood.[8] Oral lesions are usually the first sign and precede skin lesions in 50% of cases. Patients usually present with refractory lesions that can affect any mucosal surfaces. Oral mucosa is the most frequently affected mucosal site, especially the buccal mucosa, labial mucosa, palate, ventral tongue, and gingivae (**Fig. 1**). However, other mucosal surfaces such as esophageal, pharyngo-laryngeal, genital, anal, and conjunctiva may be involved.[8,10] Desquamative gingivitis is less commonly seen in PV compared with other vesiculobullous conditions.[5,10] Clinically, oral lesions appear as ragged erosions with shallow and deep ulcerations (**Figs. 2–10**). Oral lesions are

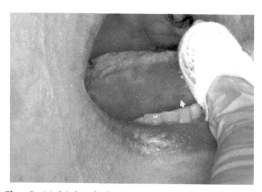

Fig. 2. Multiple shallow and deep (*arrow*) ulcers involving the right lateral border of the tongue and the left palate. The dorsal tongue appears white and thickened.

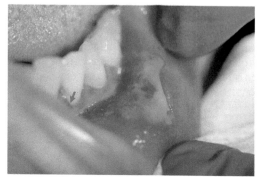

Fig. 3. Large shallow ulcer and erosion involving the lower labial mucosa. Erythematous lesions involving the marginal gingiva (*arrow*).

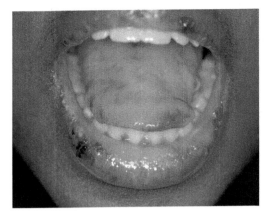

Fig. 4. Hemorrhagic and crusted lip lesions may be mistaken for erythema multiforme.

painful, often occur in posterior locations, and therefore can cause dysphagia and weight loss.[10] A positive Nikolsky's sign is a characteristic feature of PV, in which a new bulla formation can be induced on normal-appearing skin on slight lateral pressure.[3,8] The ocular lesions are uncommon, resemble conjunctivitis and unlike BMMP, and do not usually progress to scarring and symblepharon formation.[7,13]

DIAGNOSIS AND HISTOPATHOLOGIC FEATURES

Diagnosis of PV is based on the clinical scenario, histopathologic examination along with the detection of intercellular autoantibodies within the epithelium by DIF microscopy and/or circulating autoantibodies by indirect immunofluorescence (IIF), enzyme-linked immunosorbent assay (ELISA), or immunoblotting.[8,11,12]

As the lesional tissue is significantly friable and easily detached from the underlying connective tissue, a biopsy must be taken from perilesional mucosa for an accurate diagnosis.[4,6] Ulcerated and eroded mucosa should be avoided as this tissue may not be sufficient for diagnosis due to the lack of intact surface epithelium.

The classic microscopic features seen in PV are acantholysis with suprabasilar separation (**Fig. 11**A). The basal cells remain attached to the basement membrane, forming a row of tombstones appearance. Acantholysis is the result of loss of cell–cell adhesion affecting the spinous cell layer, in which large, free-floating, and rounded acantholytic epithelial cells termed "Tzanck cells" are seen.[8–12] However, the presence of Tzanck cells is not diagnostic for PV, as they can also be seen in other conditions such as herpes simplex virus infection. DIF examination is required for confirmation of the diagnosis which would reveal intercellular deposition of IgG and complement C3 in a "chicken-wire" pattern (**Fig. 11**B).[4,6–8] Circulating autoantibodies in patients' serum are typically detected in 80% to 90% of cases using IIF assay.[7,11,12]

TREATMENT AND PROGNOSIS

The prognosis of PV is highly dependent on the extent of involvement as well as early diagnosis and treatment of oral lesions before the onset of skin disease.[10,14] Oral lesions are the most difficult to resolve with treatment. Hence, the oral lesions are designated as "the first to show and the last to go."[1–5,10]

Systemic corticosteroids in combination with steroid-sparing immunosuppressant agents

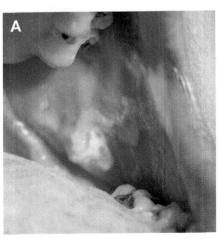
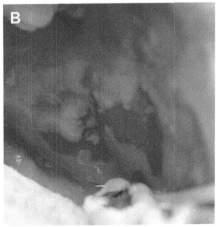

Fig. 5. (A) White plaque on the right buccal mucosa. (B) Removal of the plaque reveals erosive and erythematous mucosal surface.

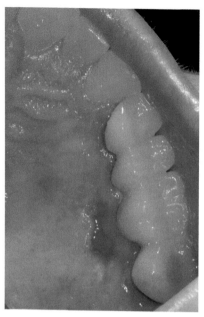

Fig. 6. Deep, well-circumscribed ulceration of the hard palate on the left side.

remain the therapeutic mainstay for pemphigus. The adjuvant immunosuppressant therapies often used are azathioprine, rituximab, methotrexate, or cyclophosphamide.[7,8,10,14]

Dexamethasone pulse therapy (DPT) has been proposed as a treatment modality for pemphigus that has been widely used. The main objective of steroid-pulse therapy is to control the disease and prevent relapses, rather than symptom alleviation.[14] The recommended DPT consists of four phases summarized in **Table 1**.

Oral lesions can benefit from combining topical corticosteroids with the systemic therapy along with maintaining great oral hygiene (**Fig. 12**). Topical corticosteroids may include clobetasol propionate ointment or gel, oral prednisolone (5 mg) dissolved in 10 to 20 mL of water and

used as a mouthwash or corticosteroid spray. These might be applied two to three times daily to aid in healing and prevent new blister formation.[8,10] In addition, appropriate antifungal therapy is recommended to prevent fungal superinfection if any.[14]

Although systemic corticosteroids are highly effective in managing the disease, long-term use may be associated with significant adverse effects, including diabetes mellitus, adrenal insufficiency, iatrogenic Cushing's syndrome, osteoporosis, peptic ulcers, and increased risk of opportunistic infections.[8,10]

PV is a chronic disease with periods of exacerbation and remission, even when patients are on treatment. Therefore, circulating autoantibodies serum levels are useful biomarkers for measuring disease activity and clinical follow-up.[8,10–12]

BENIGN MUCOUS MEMBRANE PEMPHIGOID

BMMP is a heterogeneous group of chronic, vesiculobullous autoimmune conditions, mediated essentially by IgG autoantibodies directed against different structural proteins in the basement membrane, including collagen VII, collagen XVII (also called BP180), BP230, integrin α6/β4, and laminin-332.[1–3,15–19] Collagen XVII and laminin-332 are believed to be major target antigens in BMMP. Anti-laminin-332 BMMP has been associated with an increased risk of underlying malignancies in 25% to 30% of patients.[7,20] Autoantibodies against integrin α 6/β4 have been implicated in ocular involvement.[18,20]

BMMP affects predominantly the oral, ocular mucosa and rarely, the skin.[2,15–17,19] BMMP is also called cicatricial pemphigoid derived from the word cicatrix, meaning "scar."[3] However, scarring can affect the conjunctival (ocular) mucosa only and is not seen in the oral mucosa.[3,15–17,19,21] Ocular involvement is the most significant aspect of this condition which occurs in approximately 25% of patients with oral lesions.

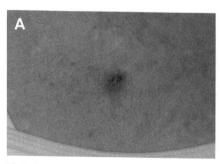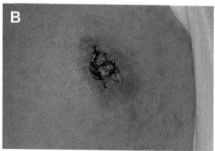

Fig. 7. (A, B) Cutaneous pemphigus vulgaris lesions. Hemorrhagic crusted ulcerations developed after bullae ruptured.

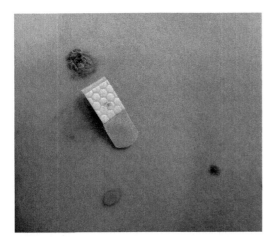

Fig. 8. Elevated, crusted, and pigmented cutaneous lesion.

Blindness may occur if the patient is not treated.[15–17,19,21]

Owing to its clinical resemblance to pemphigus, the disease is called pemphigoid or pemphigus-like. One of the most important differences with pemphigus is the type of vesicles or bullae seen in the two diseases.[7]

As the epithelial separation in pemphigus is intraepithelial compared with stronger subepithelial blisters seen in BMMP, the blisters in pemphigus are more fragile and rarely stay intact for more than a few minutes.[6,7]

CLINICAL FEATURES

BMMP is a disease of the adults and elderly and tends to affect women twice as commonly as men. Rarely, the disease has been reported in children. The average age of onset for BMMP is 60 years (range between 50 and 70 years).[15,16,19,21] Oral lesions are invariably seen (**Figs. 13–15**), but other extraoral sites, such as conjunctival, nasal, esophageal, laryngeal, and genital mucosa as well as the skin may be affected.[5,7,16,21] In two-third of the cases, the lesions are limited to the gingiva but may be seen diffusely throughout the oral mucosa. This gingival pattern of involvement is known as desquamative gingivitis (**Fig. 16**) which may also rarely be seen in other vesiculobullous conditions.[3,4,15]

Oral lesions begin as either vesicles or bullae which are durable and often filled with blood (**Fig. 17**).[3,7,15,16] The clinical finding of blood blisters is highly diagnostic of BMMP. These blisters may last for days to weeks, eventually rupturing, leaving behind superficial, ragged, and denuded areas that are usually painful and persist for weeks to months when untreated (**Fig. 17**C).[5,15,16]

Ocular involvement is the most significant complication of this disease which occurs in one-fourth of the patients with oral lesions. Usually, ocular lesions follow oral involvement.[15,16,21] The conjunctiva may become inflamed and eroded, leading to scarring between the bulbar conjunctiva of the eyeball and palpebral conjunctiva of the eyelid. As a result, adhesions (*symblepharon*) may occur (**Fig. 18**). As a protective mechanism, the cornea may produce keratin resulting in blindness.[16,21]

Laryngeal involvement is uncommon but may be especially significant because of the risk of airway obstruction by the bullae that are formed. Patients who report dysphagia, dysphonia, or dyspnea should undergo examination with laryngoscopy.[16]

DIAGNOSIS AND HISTOPATHOLOGIC FEATURES

Diagnosis of BMMP is based on the clinical findings along with the detection of tissue-bound autoantibodies by DIF microscopy and/or circulating autoantibodies by IIF, ELISA, or immunoblotting.[15,16,22]

A perilesional biopsy is recommended for reasons similar to those mentioned in the previous topic.

In H & E sections, a clear separation between the surface epithelium and the underlying

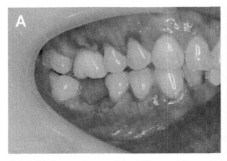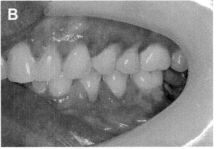

Fig. 9. (*A, B*) Multiple erosions with diffuse white, mildly thickened plaque lesions on the gingiva.

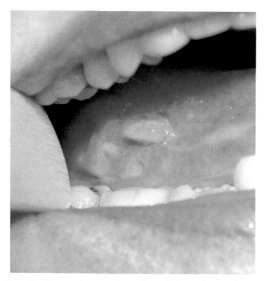

Fig. 10. Pyogenic granuloma in a sitting of pemphigus vulgaris. Hyperkeratotic and ulcerated mass arising on the right lateral border of the tongue. Note the surrounding mucosal erosions, which represent pemphigus vulgaris.

connective tissue is characteristically seen (**Fig. 19**). DIF examination is required for confirmation of the diagnosis and reveals a linear band of IgG and complement C3 deposited at the basement membrane zone (**Fig. 20**). Immunoreactivity of IgA and IgM may also be identified. One isolated study has reported that simultaneous IgG and IgA immunoreactivity may be associated with a more aggressive form of the disease.[4,15,16,22]

Unlike pemphigus, circulating autoantibodies in BMMP are usually difficult to detect and are detected in only 17% to 53% of BMMP cases using IIF assay.[16,22]

TREATMENT AND PROGNOSIS

BMMP treatment depends on the extent of involvement and severity of the disease. Mild disease usually limited to the gingiva can be treated with potent topical steroids, but once the lesions progress and especially if they involve other mucous membranes, the eyes, or the skin, then systemic therapy and referral to dermatology and/or ophthalmology are indicated. Current guidelines recommend using dapsone, methotrexate, or tetracyclines, and/or topical corticosteroids as first-line treatment.[3,4,15,16,22] For more severe cases, dapsone with systemic cyclophosphamide and/or oral corticosteroids is recommended.[15,16]

Mild to moderate oral lesions may be treated by topical corticosteroids, particularly the high-potency clobetasol propionate ointment (**Figs. 21 and 22**). Fluticasone propionate 400 μg (1 mg/mL) may also be used as a mouthwash twice daily. For severe oral lesions, dapsone with oral or topical corticosteroids is usually recommended. Systemic corticosteroids combined with dapsone and immunosuppressive agents, particularly mycophenolate mofetil, are best reserved for more severe and extensive cases.[22]

For gingival lesions, a soft medication delivery tray fabricated in the dental laboratory may be used for better contact with tissues and absorption. The custom tray should be placed in the mouth with the topical steroid in it for 10 to 12 minutes once or twice daily. Adjuvant analgesics and anti-inflammatory therapies such as chlorhexidine (0.12%–0.20%) can be used. In addition, patients

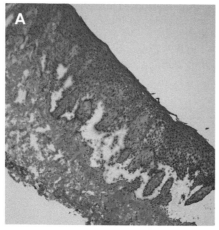
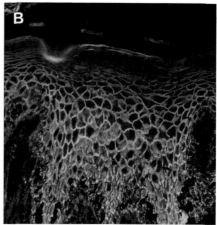

Fig. 11. (*A*) Light microscopic examination of a perilesional mucosa reveals intraepithelial separation, located just above the basal cell layer (*arrow*). (*B*) Direct immunofluorescence microscopy shows IgG deposition in intercellular spaces of the epithelial cells resulting in a network or chicken wire pattern.

Table 1
The recommended dexamethasone pulse therapy

	The Standard Dexamethasone Cyclophosphamide Pulse (DCP) Regimen	Dexamethasone Azathioprine Pulse (DAP)	Dexamethasone Methotrexate Pulse (DMP)
Phase I	Monthly doses of dexamethasone (100 mg dissolved in 500 mL of 5% dextrose) by slow intravenous infusion over 2 h on 3 consecutive days. Cyclophosphamide (500 mg) is added to the infusion on day 2. In between, low-dose oral cyclophosphamide (50 mg) and oral calcium (500 mg) daily. Vitamin D $\geq$300,000 IU once a month	Monthly doses of dexamethasone No bolus dose of azathioprine is given during the pulse. Cyclophosphamide is replaced with oral azathioprine (50 mg) daily	Monthly doses of dexamethasone No bolus dose of methotrexate is given during the pulse. Cyclophosphamide is replaced with oral methotrexate (7.5 mg, "3 doses of 2.5 mg each at 12 hourly intervals") weekly.
Phase II	Monthly dosage of DCP therapy. Low-dose oral cyclophosphamide (50 mg) and oral calcium (500 mg) daily. Continued for 9 mo, even if patients achieved complete remission. Vitamin D $\geq$ 300,000 IU once a month	Monthly dosage of DAP therapy. Oral azathioprine (50 mg) daily. Continued for 9 mo, even if patients achieved complete remission.	Monthly dosage of DMP therapy. Oral methotrexate (7.5 mg, "3 doses of 2.5 mg each at 12 hourly intervals") weekly. Continued for 9 mo, even if patients achieved complete remission.
Phase III	Continue low-dose oral Cyclophosphamide (50 mg) and oral calcium (500 mg) daily for an additional 9 mo.	Oral azathioprine (50 mg) daily for an additional 9 mo	Oral methotrexate (7.5 mg, "3 doses of 2.5 mg each at 12 hourly intervals") weekly, for an additional 9 mo.
Phase IV	Withdrawal of all treatments, and long-term follow-up for relapse if any.	Withdrawal of all treatments, and long-term follow-up for relapse if any.	Withdrawal of all treatments, and long-term follow-up for relapse if any.

with gingival involvement benefit and respond better to treatment when oral hygiene is good.[22]

Early recognition is crucial, helping to reduce disease-related morbidity and mortality and prevent life-threatening complications.

BULLOUS PEMPHIGOID

BP is the most common form of autoimmune skin blistering disease, constituting about 80% of skin autoimmune blistering cases. The estimated incidence in the United States is 6 to 13 per 1 million population diagnosed each year.[23–25]

BP is characterized by subepidermal blisters with intense generalized pruritus as well as alternating periods of remission and relapse. Most of the BP cases are mediated by autoantibodies directed against hemidesmosomes, the multiprotein structures that attach the basal epithelial cells to the basement membrane and underlying connective tissue. The target proteins (antigens) are BP antigen 1 (BPAG1, also known as Dystonin or BP230) and BP antigen 2 (BPAG2, also known as BP180 or type XVII collagen).[23–25]

A clear association of BP with certain major histocompatibility complex class II alleles, specifically

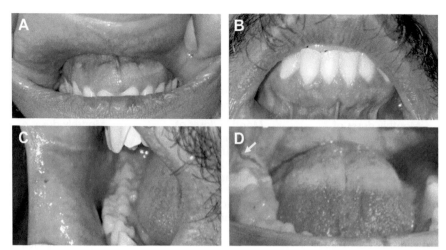

Fig. 12. Same patient as Fig. 1 after treatment with high doses of corticosteroids. (*A*) Facial maxillary gingiva. (*B*) Facial mandibular gingiva. (*C*) Scar tissue in an area of previous large ulceration of the right buccal mucosa. (*D*) Non-coated tongue, and lesion-free palatal mucosa, with only one persistent ulcer, is noted on the right mucosa (*arrow*). At this point, the patient was asymptomatic and reported weight gain.

the human leukocyte antigen class II is found in BP patients.[26]

A few cases have also been associated with certain medications. Drug-induced BP typically affects a younger subset of patients and may arise up to 3 months after initiation of the medication.[27,28] Medications most implicated in drug-induced BP are listed in **Box 1**.

CLINICAL FEATURES

BP predominantly affects elderly patients with the peak incidence in the seventh and eighth decades of life. The disease is rare in the pediatric population. BP has an equal gender distribution with no racial/ethnic predilection.[23,24] However, affected individuals may have a genetic susceptibility to developing BP.[25]

Lesions typically appear on the skin of the trunk and extremities. Usually, patients develop tense, large bullae preceded by or associated with moderate to severe pruritus, and erythematous papular eruption. However, about 20% of patients will present with pruritus without blisters at the onset of the disease. The bullae are tense, large, and range between 1 and 4 cm in diameter. They are typically filled with clear fluid but sometimes can be hemorrhagic. The duration of the bullae varies but they eventually rupture resulting in shallow ulcers, erosions, and crusts that heal without scarring. Approximately one-third of patients will have concurrent mucosal lesions.[7,23,24] Oral lesions of BP (**Fig. 23**) are similar to those of BMMP. The

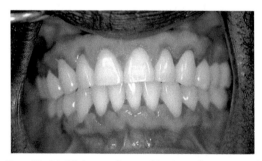

Fig. 13. Multiple erosions affecting the marginal gingiva, producing erythema and tenderness.

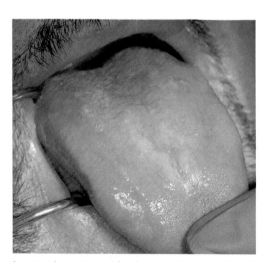

Fig. 14. Ulcerations with white striation involving the dorsal tongue resembling lichen planus.

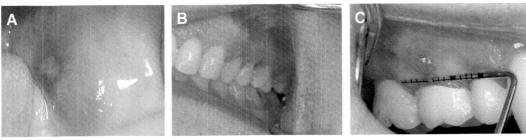

Fig. 15. (*A*) Ill-defined keratotic striae with erythematous zones and ulceration of the left buccal mucosa. (*B*) Erythematous lesion involving the left maxillary buccal vestibule. (*C*) Vesicle on the right attached gingiva that would eventually rupture, leaving raw, and painful ulceration.

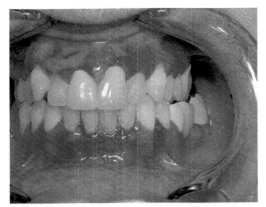

Fig. 16. Desquamative gingivitis presentation. The gingiva appears erythematous, tender, glazed, and friable.

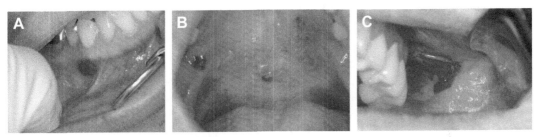

Fig. 17. (*A*) The characteristic blood-filled blister affecting the right mucogingival margin. (*B*) Multiple vesicles, and erosions on the hard and soft palate. (*C*) Raptured bulla resultant in a shallow and hemorrhagic ulcer.

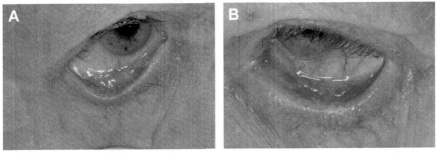

Fig. 18. (*A*) Inflamed and eroded conjunctiva. (*B*) Example of symblepharon; adhesion between the bulbar and palpebral conjunctivae.

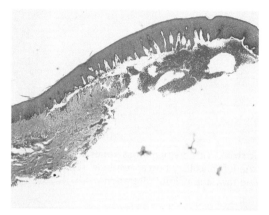

Fig. 19. Light microscopic examination of a perilesional mucosa shows a clear separation between the surface epithelium and the underlying connective tissue.

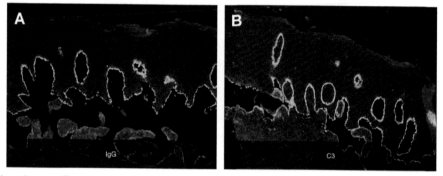

Fig. 20. Direct immunofluorescence microscopy reveals a linear band of IgG (*A*) and C3 (*B*) deposition at the basement membrane zone.

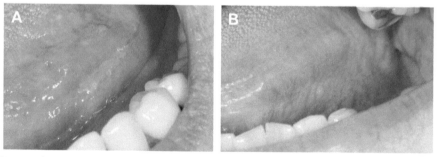

Fig. 21. (*A*) Large ulceration of the left lateral border of the tongue. (*B*) Same lesion after corticosteroids therapy. The ulceration healed completely.

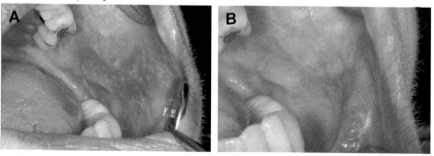

Fig. 22. (*A*) Diffuse and ill-defined erosions of the left buccal mucosa. (*B*) Near resolution of lesions after corticosteroids treatment.

<table>
<tr><td>Box 1
Medications most implicated in drug-induced
bullous pemphigoid</td></tr>
</table>

Alogliptin

Anagliptin

Aspirin

Biostim

D-Penicillamine

Enalapril

Erlotinib

Etanercept

Everolimus

Furosemide

Ibuprofen

Levofloxacin

Linagliptin

Nivolumab

Pembrolizumab

Phenacetin

Psoralens with UVA

Rifampicin

Serratiopeptidase

Sirolimus

Sitagliptin

Tetanus toxoid

Tiobutarit

Vildagliptin

DIAGNOSIS AND HISTOPATHOLOGIC FEATURES

BP diagnosis relies on the clinical findings, histologic and immunopathologic evaluations.[23–25] A biopsy must be taken from perilesional mucosa for an accurate diagnosis similar to the other entities discussed above.

Histopathologic examination of perilesional tissue demonstrates a subepithelial separation with a superficial perivascular inflammatory infiltrate and numerous eosinophils (**Fig. 24**).[3] The presence of eosinophils, especially within the bulla may provide a clue for diagnosing BP (see **Fig. 24**C). DIF studies are imperative to confirm the diagnosis. The DIF will highlight the deposition of IgG and complement C3 in a linear homogeneous pattern at the basement membrane zone similar to that seen in BMMP.[7,23–25]

Circulating autoantibodies in patients' serum are typically detected in 50% to 90% of cases using IIF assay. ELISA is also a useful diagnostic tool for BP with 89% sensitivity and 98% specificity. Several case series have shown that anti-BP180 IgG levels correlate with disease severity and could be used as a predictive marker for relapse.[30]

TREATMENT AND PROGNOSIS

BP treatment and prognosis depend on the extent of involvement and severity of the disease. However, the standard treatment is corticosteroids.[23–25] For mild disease where less than 20% of body surface area is affected, high-potency topical corticosteroids such as clobetasol propionate may be used. Combining topical corticosteroids with nicotinamide and tetracycline antibiotics (ie, doxycycline) has shown promising results in multiple cases. Systemic corticosteroids, such as prednisone at a dose of 0.5 to 1.0 mg/kg per day are reserved for more severe and extensive cases unless contraindicated.[23–25,29] Immunosuppressant therapies such as azathioprine, mycophenolate mofetil, methotrexate, and cyclophosphamide are used when systemic corticosteroids fail to control the disease. In refractory cases, intravenous immunoglobulin therapy, rituximab, or omalizumab can be used.[23–25]

Drug-induced BP cases are often self-limited and resolve spontaneously after discontinuation of the offending medication(s). Treatments are available to help relieve the symptoms and maintain quality of life.[27,28]

The disease typically has a chronic clinical course with unpredictable exacerbations. A

attached gingiva is the most frequently involved intraoral site, although the soft palate, buccal mucosa, and floor of the mouth may be affected as well.[3,29] In contrast to PV, the Nikolsky's sign is usually negative in BP.[25]

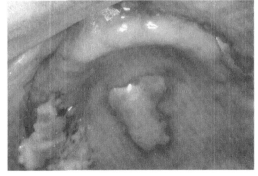

Fig. 23. Large, irregular bullae and shallow ulcerations involving the palate and the alveolar ridge.

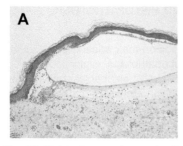
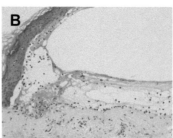
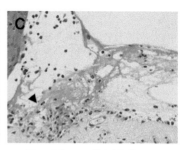

Fig. 24. Light microscopic examination reveals (A, B) a subepidermal blister with mild superficial inflammatory cell infiltrate. (C) Prominent eosinophils (*arrowhead*), a characteristic for bullous pemphigoid. (*Courtesy of* Dr Vladimir Vincek)

relapse rate of 30%-50% is observed within the first year. The mortality rate is relatively high in BP approximately 10% to 40%, mainly because it is a disease of the elderly. In addition, treatment-related adverse effects are associated with increased mortality. BP patients are susceptible to microbial infections such as varicella-zoster virus, staphylococcal, streptococcal infections, and sepsis. Patients need to avoid trauma and maintain good hygiene to prevent complications.[23–25,29]

EPIDERMOLYSIS BULLOSA ACQUISITA

Epidermolysis bullosa acquisita (EBA) is the rarest of the vesiculobullous autoimmune conditions. It is mediated by autoantibodies directed against type VII collagen, a major element of the anchoring fibrils at the stromal-epithelial junction. The estimated annual incidence of EBA is 1 case per million population., Approximately 9.6% of EBA cases have been associated with other conditions such as rheumatoid arthritis, Crohn's disease, ulcerative colitis, psoriasis, and thyroiditis. Affected individuals may have a genetic susceptibility to developing EBA.[31–36]

CLINICAL FEATURES

EBA rarely occurs in childhood, and it typically affects older adults, with an average age of 50 years and an equal gender distribution.[31–35,37] EBA is characterized by the development of blisters and bullae on the skin and mucous membranes. Mucosal involvement is seen in one-fourth of EBA cases. Oral mucosa is the most frequently affected mucosal site, followed by ocular, genital, esophageal, tracheal, and anal mucosae (**Fig. 25**). Ocular and tracheal involvement may lead to blindness and life-threatening respiratory complications, respectively, due to scarring. Atrophic scarring, hypopigmentation, onychodystrophy

(nail dystrophy), anonychia, and hand deformities may also occur (**Fig. 26**).[31–35,37,38]

Depending on EBA subtype, oral lesions can be subclinical, chronic, or severe. Usually, oral lesions are described as widespread painful blisters, erosions, and scarring that can affect any oral mucosal surfaces. In severe cases, scarring may result in ankyloglossia and trismus. Gingival involvement may manifest as gingivitis or severe periodontal disease with significant alveolar bone loss, and teeth mobility (**Fig. 27**).[38,39]

DIAGNOSIS AND HISTOPATHOLOGIC FEATURES

The International Bullous Disease Group proposed nine diagnostic criteria with a minimum of three required for EBA diagnosis (**Box 2**).[38] EBA diagnosis is established by the clinical findings, histologic and immunopathologic evaluations.[34,38] A biopsy must be taken from perilesional mucosa for an accurate diagnosis and ulcerated and eroded areas should be avoided as mentioned earlier.

Histopathologic examination of a perilesional tissue demonstrates a subepithelial/subepidermal separation with scattered inflammatory cell infiltrate (**Fig. 28**).[31–35,37,38] DIF studies are imperative

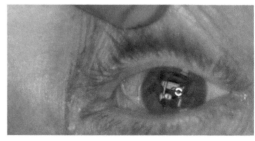

Fig. 25. Ocular involvement in epidermolysis bullosa acquisita may be mistaken for pemphigoid.

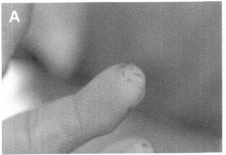 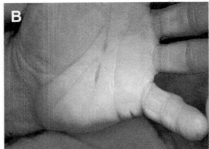

Fig. 26. Ulcerations of the fingertips (*A*) and palm (*B*).

to confirm the diagnosis. DIF highlights the deposition of IgG, complement C3, and IgA in a linear homogeneous pattern at the basement membrane zone, like that seen in BP and BMMP. However, a u-serration shaped pattern on DIF is exclusively seen in EBA and bullous systemic lupus erythematosus. This pattern differentiates EBA from pemphigoid spectrum diseases.[31–35,37,38]

IIF study on salt-split skin is a useful diagnostic tool for distinguishing EBA from BP. An artificial bulla is induced on incubated perilesional skin biopsy sample in a concentrated salt solution. When fluorescein-conjugated anti-human IgG antibodies serum is applied on the salt-split skin, in EBA cases, IgG autoantibodies will be localized to the dermal side (floor of the bulla), corresponding to collagen VII presence. This discriminates BP, where immunoreactants are localized at the epidermal side (roof of the bulla).[34,38,40]

TREATMENT AND PROGNOSIS

EBA treatment remains challenging due to the paucity of randomized controlled trials and the rarity of the disease, with most therapeutic recommendations based on small case series within the literature.

Systemic corticosteroids are used as the first line for EBA treatment. Depending on the severity and

> **Box 2**
> **International bullous disease group diagnostic criteria for the diagnosis of epidermolysis bullosa acquisita**
>
> 1. A bullous disorder within the defined clinical spectrum, *and*
> 2. Histopathology demonstrating a subepidermal or subepithelial blister (*Optional*)
> 3. Positive DIF* microscopy of perilesional tissue with linear deposition of IgG, C3, IgA, and/or IgM at the basement membrane zone, *and*
> 4. Detection of circulating anti-collagen VII autoantibodies by immunoblotting, ELISA**, and/or IIF*** microscopy on collagen VII expressing human cells, *OR*
> 5. Labeling anchoring fibrils by indirect immunoelectron microscopy or negative IIF*** microscopy on collagen VII deficient skin
>
> For seronegative patients, diagnosis is confirmed if criteria (1) *AND* (3) are present *AND* 1 or more of the following:
>
> 6. Presence of "u-serration" patterns on DIF* microscopy, *OR*
> 7. Direct immunoelectron microscopy of perilesional skin exhibiting immune deposits within anchoring fibrils zone ± sublamina densa zone, *OR*
> 8. Fluorescent overlay antigen mapping analysis showing in vivo bound immune deposits below the basal keratinocyte membrane, lamina lucida, and lamina densa components, *OR*
> 9. +Deposition of autoantibodies to the dermal side on DIF* and/or IIF*** on salt-split skin test
>
> *Direct immunofluorescence; **Enzyme-linked immunosorbent assay; ***Indirect immunofluorescence; + Can be used as an alternative to criteria (4) through (8)

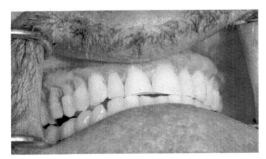

Fig. 27. Epidermolysis bullosa acquisita manifests as a periodontal disease with significant alveolar bone loss.

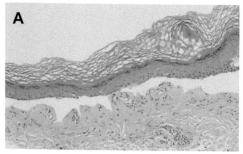 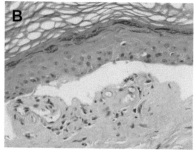

Fig. 28. (*A, B*) Light microscopic examination of a perilesional tissue demonstrates a subepidermal separation with scant inflammatory cell infiltrate. (*Courtesy of* Vladimir Vincek, MD, PhD, Gainesville, FL)

extent of the disease the initial dosage ranges from 0.5 to 2.0 mg/kg/d. Systemic corticosteroids in combination with steroid-sparing immunosuppressant therapies including dapsone, azathioprine, colchicine, cyclosporine, cyclophosphamide, methotrexate, and mycophenolate mofetil have been widely used in EBA treatment with variable success results.[31–35,37–39,41] Rituximab and high-dose intravenous Immunoglobulin have shown to be effective in EBA treatments, especially in recalcitrant cases. Despite advancements in therapy, patients may experience relapses during treatment.[41]

CLINICS CARE POINTS

- If a vesiculobullous disease is suspected the biopsy must be from unaffected, perilesional tissue

- Oral lesions in PV are the most difficult to treat and are the first to show and the last to go.

- PV starts in the oral cavity over 50% of the time and early treatment before it gets to the skin is essential

- The clinical finding of intact, persistent, blood-filled blisters is highly diagnostic of BMMP.

- Once BMMP lesions progress and especially if they involve other mucous membranes, the eyes, or the skin, then systemic therapy and referral to dermatology and/or ophthalmology is indicated.

- Bullous pemphigoid is predominantly a skin disorder with lesser oral involvement

DISCLOSURE

No financial support was provided for this work and the authors do not have conflicts of interest.

REFERENCES

1. Challacombe SJ, Setterfield JF. Oral Vesicular and Bullous Lesions. In: Farah C, Balasubramaniam R, McCullough M, editors. Contemporary oral medicine. Cham: Springer; 2018. https://doi.org/10.1007/978-3-319-28100-1_13-1.

2. Nikitakis NG. Oral Soft Tissue Lesions: A Guide to Differential Diagnosis Part II: Surface Alterations. Braz J Oral Sci 2015;4:707–15.

3. Erugula Sridhar Reddy, Kumar Singaraju Dilip, Govada Jesudass, et al. Vesiculobullous lesions of the oral cavity. IAIM 2016;3(11):154–63.

4. articleGonçalo RIC, Severo MLB, Medeiros AMC, et al. Vesiculobullous autoimmune diseases with oral mucosa manifestations: retrospective and follow-up study. Rgo, Rev Gaúch Odontol 2018; 66(1):42–9.

5. Ramos-e-Silva M, Ferreira A, Jacques Cd. Oral involvement in autoimmune bullous diseases. Clin Dermatol 2011;29(4):443–54.

6. Amagai M. Pemphigus. In: Bolognia JL, Schaffer JV, Cerroni L, editors. Dermatology. 4th edition. London: Elsevier Saunders; 2017.

7. Egami S, Yamagami J, Amagai M. Autoimmune bullous skin diseases, pemphigus and pemphigoid. J Allergy Clin Immunol 2020;145(4):1031–47.

8. Sanders WJ. A brief review of pemphigus vulgaris. Biomed Dermatol 2017;1:1–7.

9. Amagai M. Autoimmunity against desmosomal cadherins in pemphigus. J Dermatol Sci 1999;20(2): 92–102.

10. Sen S, Chakraborty R, Meshram M, et al. Oral mucosal changes in pemphigus vulgaris and its treatment: A case report. J Fam Med Prim Care 2019;8(12):4036–8.

11. Kasperkiewicz M, Ellebrecht CT, Takahashi H, et al. Pemphigus Nat Rev Dis Primers 2017;3:17026.

12. Schmidt E, Kasperkiewicz M, Joly P. Pemphigus Lancet 2019;394(10201):882–94.

13. Chirinos-Saldaña P, Zuñiga-Gonzalez I, Hernandez-Camarena JC, et al. Cicatricial changes in ocular pemphigus. Eye (Lond). 2014;28(4):459–65.

14. Mustafi S, Sinha R, Hore S, et al. Pulse therapy: Opening new vistas in treatment of pemphigus. J Fam Med Prim Care 2019;8(3):793–8.
15. Kamaguchi M, Iwata H. The Diagnosis and Blistering Mechanisms of Mucous Membrane Pemphigoid. Front Immunol 2019;10:34.
16. Chan LS, Ahmed AR, Anhalt GJ, et al. The first international consensus on mucous membrane pemphigoid: definition, diagnostic criteria, pathogenic factors, medical treatment, and prognostic indicators. Arch Dermatol 2002;138:370–9.
17. Kamaguchi M, Iwata H, Miyauchi T, et al. The identification of autoantigens in mucous membrane pemphigoid using immortalized oral mucosal keratinocytes. J Oral Pathol Med 2019;48(1):60–7.
18. Chiorean R, Danescu S, Virtic O, et al. Molecular diagnosis of anti-laminin 332 (epiligrin) mucous membrane pemphigoid. Orphanet J Rare Dis 2018;13:111.
19. Alrashdan MS, Kamaguchi M. Management of mucous membrane pemphigoid: a literature review and update [published online ahead of print, 2021 Oct 27]. Eur J Dermatol 2021. https://doi.org/10.1684/ejd.2021.4132.
20. Bernard P, Antonicelli F, Bedane C, et al. Prevalence and clinical significance of anti-laminin 332 autoantibodies detected by a novel enzyme-linked immunosorbent assay in mucous membrane pemphigoid. JAMA Dermatol 2013;149(5):533–40.
21. Morel M, DeGrazia T, Ward L, et al. Single Center Retrospective Study of Patients with Ocular Mucous Membrane Pemphigoid (MMP). Ocul Immunol Inflamm 2022;30(1):256–61.
22. Schmidt E, Rashid H, Marzano AV, et al. European Guidelines (S3) on diagnosis and management of mucous membrane pemphigoid, initiated by the European Academy of Dermatology and Venereology - Part II. J Eur Acad Dermatol Venereol 2021;35(10):1926–48.
23. Vaillant L, Bernard P, Joly P, et al. Evaluation of clinical criteria for diagnosis of bullous pemphigoid. French Bullous Study Group. Arch Dermatol 1998;134(9):1075–80.
24. Baigrie D, Nookala V. Bullous pemphigoid. StatPearls. Treasure Island (FL): StatPearls Publishing; 2021.
25. Hammers CM, Stanley JR. Mechanisms of Disease: Pemphigus and Bullous Pemphigoid. Annu Rev Pathol 2016;11:175–97.
26. Delgado JC, Turbay D, Yunis EJ, et al. A common major histocompatibility complex class II allele HLA-DQB1* 0301 is present in clinical variants of pemphigoid. Proc Natl Acad Sci U S A 1996;93(16):8569–71.
27. Verheyden MJ, Bilgic A, Murrell DF. A Systematic Review of Drug-Induced Pemphigoid. Acta Derm Venereol 2020;100(15):adv00224.
28. Stavropoulos PG, Soura E, Antoniou C. Drug-induced pemphigoid: a review of the literature. J Eur Acad Dermatol Venereol 2014;28(9):1133–40.
29. Kridin K, Bergman R. Assessment of the Prevalence of Mucosal Involvement in Bullous Pemphigoid. JAMA Dermatol 2019;155(2):166–71.
30. Mariotti F, Grosso F, Terracina M, et al. Development of a novel ELISA system for detection of anti-BP180 IgG and characterization of autoantibody profile in bullous pemphigoid patients. Br J Dermatol 2004;151(5):1004–10.
31. Roenigk HH Jr, Ryan JG, Bergfeld WF. Epidermolysis bullosa acquisita. Report of three cases and review of all published cases. Arch Dermatol 1971;103(1):1–10.
32. Gammon WR, Briggaman RA, Woodley DT, et al. Epidermolysis bullosa acquisita–a pemphigoid-like disease. J Am Acad Dermatol 1984;11(5 Pt 1):820–32.
33. Ludwig RJ. Clinical presentation, pathogenesis, diagnosis, and treatment of epidermolysis bullosa acquisita. ISRN Dermatol 2013;2013:812029.
34. Kridin K, Kneiber D, Kowalski EH, et al. Epidermolysis bullosa acquisita: A comprehensive review. Autoimmun Rev 2019;18(8):786–95.
35. Miyamoto D, Gordilho JO, Santi CG, et al. Epidermolysis bullosa acquisita. An Bras Dermatol 2022;97(4):409–23.
36. Zumelzu C, Le Roux-Villet C, Loiseau P, et al. Black patients of African descent and HLA-DRB1*15:03 frequency overrepresented in epidermolysis bullosa acquisita. J Invest Dermatol 2011;131(12):2386–93.
37. Iwata H, Vorobyev A, Koga H, et al. Meta-analysis of the clinical and immunopathological characteristics and treatment outcomes in epidermolysis bullosa acquisita patients. Orphanet J Rare Dis 2018;13(1):153.
38. Prost-Squarcioni C, Caux F, Schmidt E, et al. International Bullous Diseases Group: consensus on diagnostic criteria for epidermolysis bullosa acquisita. Br J Dermatol 2018;179(1):30–41.
39. Marzano AV, Cozzani E, Fanoni D, et al. Diagnosis and disease severity assessment of epidermolysis bullosa acquisita by ELISA for anti-type VII collagen autoantibodies: an Italian multicentre study. Br J Dermatol 2013;168(1):80–4.
40. Lazarova Z, Yancey KB. Reactivity of autoantibodies from patients with defined subepidermal bullous diseases against 1 mol/L salt-split skin. Specificity, sensitivity, and practical considerations. J Am Acad Dermatol 1996;35(3 Pt 1):398–403.
41. Kasperkiewicz M, Sadik CD, Bieber K, et al. Epidermolysis Bullosa Acquisita: From Pathophysiology to Novel Therapeutic Options. J Invest Dermatol 2016;136(1):24–33.

Ulcerative and Inflammatory Lesions of the Oral Mucosa

Elizabeth M. Philipone, DMD*, Scott M. Peters, DDS

KEYWORDS

- Traumatic ulcers • Foreign body reactions • Necrotizing sialometaplasia • Geographic tongue
- Thermal and chemical injuries • Lesions associated with chemo and/or radiation therapy
- Drug abuse • Oral piercings and dermal fillers

KEY POINTS

- The causes of ulcerations and inflammatory lesions of the oral mucosa are variable and include mechanical, chemical, thermal, and ischemic injuries, as well as foreign body reactions.
- A detailed and careful review of the patient's history and symptoms is crucial in rendering an accurate clinical diagnosis or differential diagnoses.
- Biopsy is indicated for oral ulcerations or inflammation that fails to resolve and/or to confirm the clinical diagnosis.

CONTENT

Traumatic Ulcers

Traumatic ulcers (TUs) are a relatively common in the oral cavity. TUs can be either acute or chronic. Acute TUs are characteristically painful and have a yellow-tan base and an erythematous halo. Acute ulcers will resolve in 7 to 10 days if the cause is eliminated. Chronic oral ulcers, however, persist greater than 2 weeks, elicit little to no pain, have a yellow-tan center, and demonstrate white, elevated and/or keratotic margins (**Fig. 1**). On palpation, chronic TUs can feel indurated. This firmness is the result of chronic inflammatory infiltration and subsequent fibrosis.[1]

Traumatic ulcerative granuloma with stromal eosinophilia (TUGSE) is a specific type of chronic ulcer in which the inflammation extends into the underlying muscle. Clinically it most often occurs on the lateral tongue and presents as a long-standing, indurated ulcer with raised or rolled borders (**Fig. 2**). Microscopically, it demonstrates a lymphocytic and eosinophilic inflammatory infiltrate that extends into the underlying skeletal muscle.[2]

The clinical presentation of chronic TUs, particularly TUGSE, can mimic other conditions including squamous cell carcinoma, syphilitic chancre, and deep fungal infection. It is for this reason that biopsy is recommended for all oral ulcers that persist more than 2 weeks despite the removal of any identifiable inciting factor (ie, a sharp tooth cusp).[3] In some cases, a cause for the traumatic ulcer cannot be identified and in rare cases may be factitial. TUs often have sharp(-geometric) borders.

Most TUs will resolve on their own and should remain under observation until they heal. Topical corticosteroids such as lidex or clobetasol 0.05% gels can help hasten healing and reduce pain. Intralesional corticosteroid injections might be beneficial for TUGSE.[2]

Foreign Body Reactions

Foreign body reactions occur when exogenous material becomes embedded within oral mucosal tissues. There is an associated inflammatory response, during which the body attempts to wall off the foreign material. This results in a pattern

Division of Oral and Maxillofacial Pathology, Columbia University Irving Medical Center, New York, NY 10032, USA
* Corresponding author.
E-mail address: ep2464@cumc.columbia.edu

Oral Maxillofacial Surg Clin N Am 35 (2023) 219–226
https://doi.org/10.1016/j.coms.2022.10.001
1042-3699/23/© 2022 Elsevier Inc. All rights reserved.

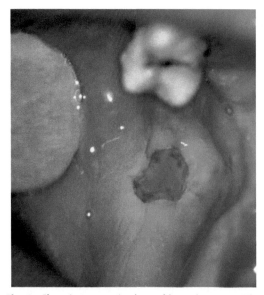

Fig. 1. Chronic traumatic ulcer of buccal mucosa. The ulcer is depressed with well-defined borders. Portions of the border seem keratotic. Note that the patient also has leukoedema.

of granulomatous inflammation when the lesion is examined microscopically.[4] Foreign body reactions may have varied clinical presentations. If particulate foreign matter is deposited in the gingiva, the gingiva will become inflamed, erythematous, and hyperplastic. This may occur infrequently following the use of certain brands of dental ultrasonic scalers and is termed granulomatous gingivitis (**Fig. 3**).[5] Foreign body reactions may also

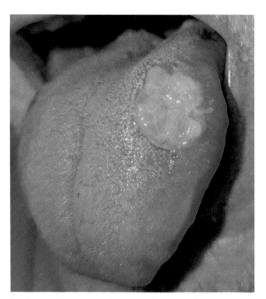

Fig. 2. TUGSE presenting as a chronic ulceration with a tan center and elevated margins.

present as poor or nonhealing ulcerations or raised nodular masses resembling more frequently encountered benign, reactive pathologic conditions. This latter presentation is often how oral lesions associated with dermal fillers will present. A foreign body reaction may be considered in the clinical differential diagnosis based on provided patient history; however, a biopsy of the lesion is required to confirm the diagnosis. Microscopic examination will demonstrate granulomatous inflammation and polarizable foreign material. The absence of identifiable foreign material does not necessarily preclude this diagnosis; however, other causes of granulomatous inflammation such as tuberculosis, sarcoidosis, Crohn disease, and systemic fungal infections need to be excluded.[6]

Necrotizing Sialometaplasia

Necrotizing sialometaplasia is a benign but clinically worrisome tumor-like lesion most frequently affecting the minor salivary glands of the palate. Reactive and inflammatory in nature, the lesion initially presents as a localized soft tissue swelling in which the mucosa then sloughs resulting in a crater-like ulcer (**Fig. 4**). Necrotizing sialometaplasia is thought to be the result of localized ischemic necrosis. Causes for the ischemia include but are not limited to trauma, local anesthetic injection, smoking, and bulimia.[7] Lesions are typically a few centimeters in diameter. Most are unilateral although bilateral lesions have been reported.[8,9] Surprisingly most patients do not complain of pain despite their clinical appearance. The clinical presentation can mimic squamous cell carcinoma or a salivary gland tumor. Biopsy is indicated to confirm the diagnosis.

Microscopically, as the name implies, necrotizing sialometaplasia demonstrates necrosis of the minor salivary acinar structures and squamous metaplasia of the ducts in a background of chronic inflammation and fibrosis. It can also show psuedoepitheliomatous hyperplasia of the surface epithelium. These surface and ductal epithelial changes can be misinterpreted by the pathologist as squamous cell or mucoepidermoid carcinoma.[9]

Necrotizing sialometaplasia heals on its own during the course of several weeks.

Geographic Tongue

Geographic tongue, also referred to as benign migratory glossitis or erythema migrans, is a commonly encountered variation of normal anatomy. It can be detected in approximately 1% to 3% of the population, with no strong race, gender, or age predilection.[10] It most commonly involves

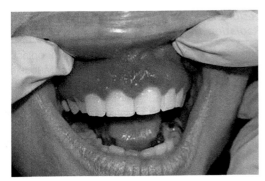

Fig. 3. Granulomatous gingivitis presenting as inflamed, hyperplastic, and erythematous gingiva. Biopsy of the tissue confirmed the presence of granulomatous inflammation.

the tongue and presents as one or multiple flat, erythematous, depapillated areas surrounded by yellow-white serpiginous borders (**Fig. 5**). The anterior and dorsal aspects of the tongue are most often affected; however, the lesions may also involve the lateral and ventral tongue surfaces. Geographic tongue is seen more frequently in patients who have fissured tongue.[11] These lesions may also occasionally be seen on other oral mucosal sites, such as the labial mucosa, buccal mucosa, and palatal mucosa (**Fig. 6**). In these instances, the terms benign migratory stomatitis or ectopic geographic tongue may be used. Areas of geographic tongue will characteristically disappear and subsequently reappear, and their clinical appearance with regard to affected site and number of lesions may vary from day to day. Geographic tongue can be diagnosed based on the clinical appearance of the lesions but if a biopsy is performed, it will demonstrate features similar to those of psoriasis (psoriasiform mucositis) and show collections of neutrophils within the spinous layers of the epithelium (Munro

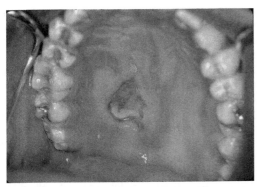

Fig. 4. Necrotizing sialometaplasia resulting in a crater-like ulcer.

microabscesses).[12] No treatment of asymptomatic geographic tongue is indicated because it represents a benign variation of normal anatomy. A small percentage of patients with geographic tongue will experience discomfort such as a burning, stinging, or itching sensation exacerbated by spicy, acidic, and/or citrus-based foods and beverages.[10] This is most appropriately managed with topical steroid therapy as needed for symptomatic flare-ups. Symptomatic geographic tongue should be ruled out in patients being evaluated for burning mouth syndrome.

Thermal and Chemical Injuries

Minor thermal and chemical injuries to the oral mucosa are not infrequent. Fortunately, serious thermal and chemical injuries are rare.

Thermal injuries are often the result of consuming too hot food and beverages. Microwave heated food is the most common offender. High temperatures produce a scalding of the mucosal tissue, which can develop into vesicles and ulcers[13] (**Fig. 7**). Besides food and beverages, oral thermal burns from the explosion of e-cigarettes, reverse smoking, and smoking of crack cocaine have been reported. Iatrogenic thermal burns can also occur in the dental office. Overheated electric handpieces,[14] lasers and heated border molding material are some possible offenders.

For treatment, if the burn is not severe, it will heal on its own within 2 weeks. Application of topical corticosteroid and local anesthetic can be helpful. For severe burns, necrotic tissue should be debrided in order to hasten granulation tissue formation and allow for healing.[15]

Chemical injuries are caused by contact with acidic or alkaline substances (**Fig. 8**). Minor chemical injuries commonly result from the use of oral dentifrices (ie, alcohol-based or peroxide-containing mouthwashes). Other more serious chemical injury can be the result of cocaine and/or methylenedioxymethamphetamine use.[13] Oral chemical burns can also occur in the dental setting because the use of caustic solutions is not uncommon. For example, mucosal contact with sodium hypochlorite during root canal irrigation results in significant tissue damage.

As soon as chemical contact has occurred the site should be irrigated. Most superficial chemical injuries will resolve without treatment within 2 weeks. The use of a topical emollient paste or dressing with a hydroxypropyl cellulose film can be beneficial.[15] Topical anesthetics or over-the-counter analgesics can be used for pain relief if warranted. The treatment of more severe chemical

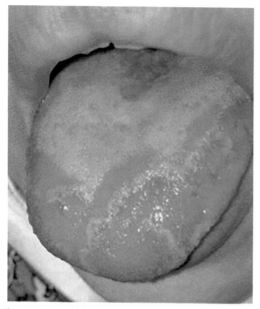

Fig. 5. Geographic tongue involving the dorsal aspect of the tongue.

injuries depends on whether the injury was caused by an acid or base. Damage caused by acidic chemicals tends to remain more superficial and can be treated as outlined above. Damage caused by alkaline chemicals, such as sodium hypochlorite, tends to extend deeper into the tissue and often requires debridement.[15]

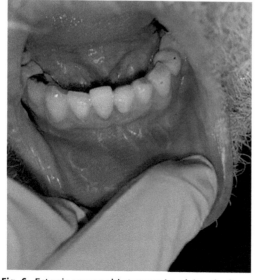

Fig. 6. Ectopic geographic tongue involving the lower labial mucosa.

Lesions Associated with Chemo and/or Radiation Therapy

The most serious complication of antineoplastic therapy in the oral cavity is mucositis. Mucositis may result from either high-dose chemotherapy or head and neck radiation in which the radiation field includes part or all of the oral cavity. Oral mucositis occurs several days to weeks after the offending medication or radiation treatment is administered. The affected mucosa will initially develop a whitish color. This whitish material subsequently desquamates, and the mucosa then seems erythematous and inflamed. In some cases, large ulcerations with overlying yellowish fibrino-purulent membranes will form (**Fig. 9**).[16] Oral mucositis is exceedingly painful, and patients will often report difficulty eating, drinking, and speaking. Treatment options for oral mucositis are limited, and preventative measures such as cryotherapy and limiting the dosage and/or field of radiation, if possible, are recommended.[16] If the field of radiation includes the salivary glands, xerostomia becomes another complication of head and neck radiation treatment. Xerostomia results from destruction of the salivary glands, which are particularly radiosensitive. Saliva acts both as a lubricant and a protective buffer, and a decrease in salivary output results in higher rates of dental caries and traumatic lesions of the oral soft tissues. In cases of severe xerostomia, the mucosa may seem cracked and atrophied. Patients with xerostomia may also report difficulty swallowing and altered taste sensations. Xerostomia can be treated with sialogogue therapy; however, patients will often experience only transient improvement in symptoms.[17] Radiation therapy and chemotherapy may also affect the jawbones. Osteoradionecrosis is defined as exposed nonvital irradiated bone, which has been present for 3 months in the absence of any local neoplastic disease. Osteoradionecrosis is seen in patients who received head and neck radiation doses of greater than 60 Gy.[18] The mandible is involved much more frequently than the maxilla. Medication-induced osteonecrosis of the jaw (MRONJ) may result from antineoplastic or antiresorptive medications used in the treatment of conditions such as multiple myeloma, breast cancer, and prostate cancer. MRONJ is defined as exposed nonvital bone for greater than 8 weeks in the setting of previous or current antiresorptive or antiangiogenic therapies and in the absence of any neoplastic disease or history or radiation therapy to the head and neck.[18] Both osteoradionecrosis and MRONJ will present as variably painful areas of yellow-tan exposed bone (**Fig. 10**). Radiographic examination

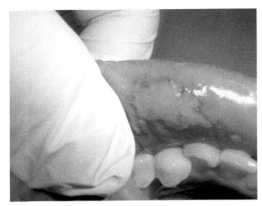

Fig. 7. Superficial ulcerations of the lower lip mucosa from thermal injury.

will demonstrate ill-defined radiolucencies with some radiopaque bony sequestra. MRONJ can often be distinguished from radiation-related osteonecrosis by the localization of the necrosis to the alveolar process. On microscopic examination, both osteoradionecrosis and MRONJ will show nonvital bone exhibiting loss of osteocytes from the lacunae surrounded by inflammatory cells and bacterial debris. Some chemotherapeutic agents may also cause pigmented lesions of the oral mucosa. This is discussed in greater detail in Chapter 11.

Oral Lesions Associated with Drug Abuse

Drug abuse is a serious problem in the United States. According to the National Center for Drug Abuse Statistics, as of 2020, just greater than 37 million Americans were current illegal drug users.

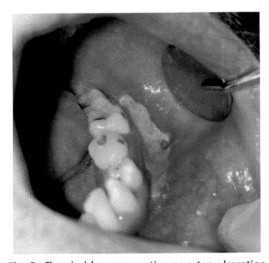

Fig. 8. Chemical burn presenting as a tan ulceration of the vestibule caused by patient's use of undiluted hydrogen peroxide.

The type of oral lesions associated with drug abuse depends on the type of drug and how it is consumed. The drugs covered in this section include cannabis, cocaine, amphetamine, and opiates. Cannabis is commonly mixed with tobacco and smoked. Cocaine is snorted; however, it can be injected or smoked in the form of crack. Amphetamines can be inhaled, injected, smoked, ingested in pill form, or dissolved in a liquid. Opioids can be taken in pill form or the pill can be crushed and snorted or injected.[19]

Regardless of the particular drug or method of abuse, addicts often demonstrate poor oral hygiene, rampant tooth decay, periodontal disease, xerostomia, and candidiasis. In addition, oral leukoplakia and squamous cell carcinoma have been associated with *smoking* cannabis.[20] Cocaine/crack when inhaled can lead to perforation of the nasal septum and palate (**Fig. 11**). Smoking of crack and methamphetamine can result in lip and mucosal burns as discussed previously. Methamphetamine has a direct eroding effect on the mouth due to its acidity, which contributes to characteristic "meth mouth" and severe xerostomia (**Fig. 12**). Self-inflicted injuries to the mucosa and facial skin also occur in relation to drug abuse.[19,21] Methamphetamine use can trigger formication—hallucinations of bugs crawling on the skins—which induces itching and scratching and resultant ulceration and tissue destruction.

Abusers often use more than one drug and are at increased risk for untoward sequelae. Intravenous users are also at the risk of infectious diseases such as HIV and hepatitis.[19,21] Psychosis and paranoia associated with drug abuse can interfere with providing dental care. Local anesthetic with a vasoconstrictor can put patients on methamphetamines and cocaine at increased risk for a hypertensive crisis. Combining opioids and benzodiazepines can increase the risk of fatal respiratory suppression.[21]

Lesions Associated with Oral Sex

Although the dental provider should be cognizant of the oral manifestations of sexually transmitted illnesses, this section focuses on oral lesions caused by physical injuries resulting from oral sex. Oral sex may result in palatal petechiae, which is typically asymptomatic and should resolve spontaneously after a few days (**Fig 13**).[22] In patients with larger, nonresolving erythematous or purple-colored lesions of the palate, conditions such as chronic cough or recent physical trauma should be considered as well.[23] Kaposi sarcoma should be excluded also

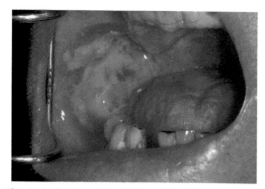

Fig. 9. Radiation mucositis involving the buccal mucosa, palate, and dorsal tongue.

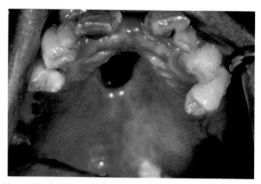

Fig. 11. Palatal perforation secondary to inhaled cocaine abuse.

especially in patients with a known history of immune compromise (HIV/AIDS, status posttransplant). Oral sex can also cause ulceration, irritation/hyperkeratosis/leukoplakia, and occasionally fibrous hyperplasia of the lingual frenum. This results from stretching of the tongue and irritation of this site against the mandibular incisor teeth.[24] An ulceration at this site will resolve spontaneously if repeated irritation does not occur. If ulcers/leukoplakia persists, a biopsy is indicated as a type of human papilloma virus (HPV)-induced severe koilocytic dysplasia has recently been described with increased frequency at this site. If fibrous hyperplasia of the frenum develops, it will clinically resemble a fibroma and is best managed via either continued observation or excisional biopsy.

Lesions Associated with Piercings

Oral and perioral piercing has historically been practiced in certain groups for religious, tribal, or cultural reasons. Currently, in the United States,

oral and perioral piercings are popular in teens and young adults. These piercings can result in several acute and chronic sequelae. Acute complications from piercings include bleeding, swelling, allergic reactions, and infection. Not surprisingly, due to the microbial environment of the mouth, infections are a common complication of oral/perioral piercing.[25] Endocarditis has even been reported as a complication from tongue piercings.[26]

Chronic lesions including mucoceles, hyperplastic scarring, traumatic fibromas, pyogenic granulomas and granulomatous inflammation are among the reported sequela.[25] Frictional irritation and repetitive trauma from the jewelry can cause mucosal abrasions, ulcerations, and gingival recession.

Hard tissue changes from trauma can result in bone loss and dehiscence and chipped and fractured teeth.[27]

Oral Lesions Associated with Dermal Fillers

The frequency of oral lesions caused by dermal (cosmetic) fillers is steadily increasing, due in large part to the increase in dermal filler use during

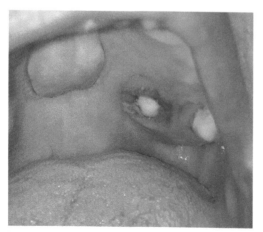

Fig. 10. Osteoradionecrosis of the maxilla in a patient with a history of head and neck radiation.

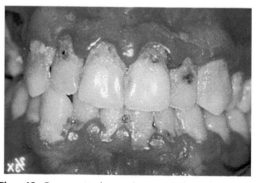

Fig. 12. Rampant decay in a methamphetamine abuser.

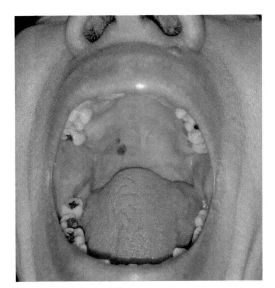

Fig. 13. Palatal petechiae.

recent years. Once limited to plastic surgery practices, treatment with dermal fillers is now being performed by general dentists, oral and maxillofacial surgeons, dermatologists, and sometimes illicitly by those without proper medical training. Adverse reactions to dermal fillers may present as lines or ridges caused by improper deposition technique or nodules may seem caused by clumping of the filler material. In some instances, these lesions may develop at a site remote from where the filler was administered due to dislocation of the material by muscle activity. Dermal fillers often cause foreign body reactions resulting in granuloma formation and desired edema.[28] Dermal fillers are derived from either natural or synthetic materials. Natural fillers, such as calcium hydroxyapatite, poly-L-lactic acid, and hyaluronic acid, are biological substrates, which can be degraded by enzymatic and phagocytic activities. These natural fillers are therefore safer to administer, although their effects are more short-lived. Synthetic fillers, however, are nonbiodegradable and therefore more prone to adverse reactions. The brand of filler material used can often be ascertained by histologic analysis of the lesion because the microscopic appearance of the foreign body reaction will vary based on dermal filler type.[28] Clinically, oral lesions associated with dermal fillers most often involve the labial mucosa, the vestibular mucosa, or the anterior buccal mucosa. They present as inert tumor-like nodules resembling more frequently encountered reactive mucosal pathologic conditions such as fibromas, lipomas, or mucoceles. In many instances, a dermal filler reaction will not be considered in the clinical differential diagnosis because the patient will often not disclose a history of filler treatment, and the diagnosis is made only on microscopic examination.[29] This biopsy is often excisional in nature and serves as definitive treatment of most lesions. Rarely, dermal filler use will result in vascular compromise from either intravascular injection of a dermal filler or arterial compression following filler injection. These episodes are exceedingly rare but can cause significant tissue ischemia and necrosis.[30]

CLINICS CARE POINTS

- The clinical presentation of oral ulcers, particularly TUGSE, can mimic other conditions including squamous cell carcinoma, syphilitic chancre, and deep fungal ulcer.
- Biopsy is recommended for oral ulcers that persist more than 2 weeks despite the removal of any identifiable inciting factor.
- Foreign body reactions may have varied clinical presentations including erythematous and hyperplastic mucosa, nonhealing ulcerations, or raised nodular masses.
- The clinical presentation of necrotizing sialometaplasia can mimic squamous cell carcinoma or a salivary gland tumor.
- Geographic tongue is detected in approximately 1% to 3% of the population and is considered a variation of normal anatomy.
- Damage caused by alkaline chemicals, such as sodium hypochlorite, tends to extend deep into the tissue and often requires debridement.

REFERENCES

1. Regezi JA, Scuibba JJ, Jordan RCK. Oral pathology : clinical pathologic correlations. 6th edition. St. Louis, Mo: Elsevier/Saunders; 2012. p. 22–6.
2. Lakkam BD, Astekar M, Alam S, et al. Traumatic ulcerative granuloma with stromal eosinophilia: A puzzle. J Oral Maxillofac Pathol 2021 Mar;25(Suppl 1): S42–5.
3. Avon SL, Klieb HB. Oral soft-tissue biopsy: an overview. J Can Dent Assoc 2012;78.c75.
4. Koh RU, Ko E, Oh TJ, et al. Foreign body gingivitis. J Mich Dent Assoc 2015;97(3):44–7.
5. Terry MA, Narayana N, Kaldahl W. Gingival foreign body granuloma in conjunction with the use of a dental water jet: a case report. Gen Dent 2014; 62(5):37–9.

6. Alawi F. Granulomatous diseases of the oral tissues: differential diagnosis and update. Dent Clin North AM 2005;49(1):203–21.

7. Carlson DL, May. Necrotizing sialometaplasia: a practical approach to the diagnosis. Arch Pathol Lab Med 2009;133(5):692–8.

8. Krishna S. Necrotizing sialometaplasia of palate: a case report. Imaging Sci Dent 2011;41(1):35–8.

9. Brannon RB, Fowler CB, Hartman KS. Necrotizing sialometaplasia. A clinicopathologic study of sixty-nine cases and review of the literature. Oral Surg Oral Med Oral Pathol 1991;72:317–25.

10. Gonzalez-Alvarez L, Garcia-Pola MJ, Garcia-Martin JM. Geographic tongue: Predisposing factors, diagnosis and treatment. A systematic review. Rev Clin Esp (Barc) 2018;218(9):481–8.

11. Zargari O. The prevalence and significance of fissured tongue and geographical tongue in psoriatic patients. Clin Exp Dermatol 2006;31:192–5.

12. Picciani BL, Domingos TA, Teixeira-Souza T, et al. Geographic tongue and psoriasis: clinical, histopathological, immunohistochemical and genetic correlation–a literature review. An Bras Dermatol 2016;91(4):410–21.

13. Guerrieri POliveira A, Arosio F, Vigano L, et al. Chemical, thermal and electrical lesions in the oral cavity. Curr Anal Dentistry 2019;2:1–4.

14. Sarrett DC. A laboratory evaluation of electric handpiece temperature and the associated risk of burns. ADA Prof Prod Rev 2014;9(2):18–24.

15. Kang S, Kufta K, Sollecito TP, et al. A treatment algorithm for the management of intraoral burns: a narrative review. Burns 2018;44(5):1065–76.

16. Lalla RV, Saunders DP, Peterson DE. Chemotherapy or radiation-induced oral mucositis. Dent Clin North Am 2014;58(2):341–9.

17. Chambers MS, Rosenthal DI, Weber RS. Radiation-induced xerostomia. Head Neck 2007;29(1):58–63.

18. Akashi M, Wanifuchi S, Iwata E, et al. Differences between osteoradionecrosis and medication-related osteonecrosis of the jaw. Oral Maxillofac Surg 2018;22(1):59–63.

19. Teoh L, Moses G, McCullough MJ. Oral manifestations of illicit drug use. Aust Dent J 2019;64(3): 213–22.

20. Cho CM, Hirsch R, Johnstone S. General and oral health implications of cannabis use. Aust Dent J 2005;50:70–4.

21. Nack B, Haas SE, Portnof J. Opioid use disorder in dental patients: the latest on how to identify, treat, refer and apply laws and regulations in your practice. Anesth Prog 2017;64(3):178–87.

22. Damm DD, White DK, Brinker CM. Variations of palatal erythema secondary to fellatio. Oral Surg Oral Med Oral Pathol 1981;52:417–21.

23. Terezhalmy GT. Oral manifestations of sexually related diseaes. Ear Nose Throat J 1983;62:287–96.

24. Mader CL. Lingual frenum ulcer resulting from orogenital sex. J Am Dent Assoc 1981;103:888–90.

25. Escudero-Castaño N, Perea-García MA, Campo-Trapero J, et al. Oral and perioral piercing complications. Open Dent J 2008;2:133–6.

26. Friedel JM, Stehlik J, Desai M, et al. Infective endocarditis after oral body piercing. Cardiol Rev 2003; 11(5):252–5.

27. De Urbiola Alís I, Viñals Iglesias H. Some considerations about oral piercings. Av Odontoestomatol 2005;21(5):259–69.

28. Owosho AA, Bilodeau EA, Vu J, et al. Orofacial dermal fillers: foreign body reactions, histopathologic features, and spectrometric studies. Oral Surg Oral Med Oral Path Oral Radiol 2014;117(5):617–25.

29. Tamiolakis P, Piperi E, Christopoulos P, et al. Oral foreign body granuloma to soft tissue fillers. Report of two cases and review of the literature. J Clin Exp Dent 2018;10(2):e177–84.

30. Halepas S, Peters SM, Goldsmith JL, et al. Vascular compromise after soft tissue facial fillers: Case report and review of current treatment protocols. J Oral Maxillofac Surg 2020;78(3):440–5.

Oral Lesions Associated with Systemic Disease

Jasbir D. Upadhyaya, BDS, MSc, PhD[a],*, Vimi Sunil Mutalik, BDS, MDS, MS, FRCD(C)[b]

KEYWORDS

- Systemic disease • Oral manifestations • Ulcerations • Cobblestone • Xerostomia

KEY POINTS

- Oral manifestations may be the first, and sometimes the only, sign of a systemic disease.
- Some conditions have characteristic features that allow for early detection, whereas others require a comprehensive dental and medical evaluation to establish a definitive diagnosis.
- Identification of oral manifestations can allow for early diagnosis and intervention in patients with systemic diseases.

INTRODUCTION

Many systemic diseases are accompanied by oral manifestations. Several studies have documented an association between periodontal disease and systemic conditions, such as cardiovascular disease and diabetes mellitus.[1–3] Oral manifestations may be the first sign of a systemic disease or may represent a recurrent or refractory disease. Many diseases present with clinically similar oral lesions and require an extensive workup to establish a diagnosis. Oral ulceration, for example, may be a sign of lupus erythematosus, pemphigus vulgaris, Behçet disease, Crohn's disease (CD), and many syndromic conditions. Generalized gingival enlargement should prompt investigation for conditions like hyperplastic gingivitis, drug-related gingival hyperplasia, gingival fibromatosis, leukemia, Wegener granulomatosis, and nutritional deficiencies like scurvy. Severe gingival inflammation may be seen in diabetes mellitus, human immunodeficiency virus infection, leukemia, and thrombocytopenia. Therefore, a comprehensive examination of the oral cavity and a thorough history taking can aid in determining the underlying etiology of oral lesions and allow for early diagnosis and intervention. The present article provides a succinct review of oral manifestations of select systemic diseases.

AMYLOIDOSIS
Description

Amyloidosis is a rare condition characterized by the extracellular deposition of insoluble amyloid fibrils, a material formed from protein misfolding. There are 30 human fibrillary proteins and each type of amyloidosis is associated with a specific protein.[4] The common forms include: *AL,* which can occur alone or in association with multiple myeloma and is caused by deposition of monoclonal immunoglobulin light chains; *AA,* which develops as a result of chronic diseases such as rheumatoid arthritis, tuberculosis, sarcoidosis; $A\beta_2M$ is associated with long-term renal dialysis. Some forms are inherited and known as heredofamilial amyloidosis.

Clinical Features

Deposition of amyloid may be localized or diffuse. Any site in the head and neck region can be affected, however, the larynx is the most common site for amyloid deposition.[5] The most frequently

[a] Department of Applied Dental Medicine, Southern Illinois University School of Dental Medicine, 2800 College Avenue, Building 285, Alton, IL 62002, USA; [b] Department of Dental Diagnostic and Surgical Sciences, University of Manitoba Dr. Gerald Niznick College of Dentistry, 780 Bannatyne Avenue, Winnipeg, Manitoba R3E 0W2, Canada
* Corresponding author.
E-mail address: jupadhy@siue.edu

Oral Maxillofacial Surg Clin N Am 35 (2023) 227–236
https://doi.org/10.1016/j.coms.2022.10.002
1042-3699/23/Published by Elsevier Inc.

reported intraoral location is the tongue, and amy-loid deposition may result in macroglossia.[6] Amyloidosis of the head and neck sites, excluding the larynx, is usually associated with an underlying condition.[7] As amyloidosis is often associated with nonspecific signs and symptoms, such as fatigue, and weight loss, the diagnosis is often rendered after a biopsy is performed. Patients may exhibit yellowish, red, or purplish papules, individual nod-ules or diffuse swelling, submucosal hemorrhage, or ulcerations of the oral mucosa.[6] The tongue is often enlarged, firm to rubbery on palpation, and typically shows scalloping of the lateral borders due to indentations from the teeth (**Fig. 1**A). Amy-loid deposits in the upper aerodigestive tract can cause hoarseness and dysphagia.[5] Systemic manifestations arise from the deposition of amy-loid in various tissues that results in heart failure, nephrotic syndrome, hepatomegaly, and periph-eral or autonomic neuropathy. Infiltration of the salivary and lacrimal glands may cause xerosto-mia and dry eyes. Skin lesions manifest as subcu-taneous plaques or nodules. Amyloid infiltration of the blood vessels increases vessel fragility result-ing in submucosal hemorrhage that manifests as purpura, petechiae, and ecchymosis in the perior-bital areas (**Fig. 1**B).

Histopathology

Amyloid seems as an amorphous, acellular, eosin-ophilic material in the submucosal connective tis-sue that may be either diffusely distributed or arranged in a perivascular manner. Amyloid stains with Congo-red and under polarized light shows an apple-green birefringence.

Diagnosis and Management

Biopsy of rectal mucosa and subcutaneous abdominal fat tissue is typically used to confirm the diagnosis.[8] Gingiva and labial salivary glands are potential sites for intraoral biopsy.[6] After confirmation of diagnosis, it is important to identify the type of amyloidosis because different forms of amyloid proteins lead to substantially different prognoses and outcomes.[5] Patients should be referred to a hematologist, and a comprehensive workup should be performed for the evaluation of systemic disorders. Treatment is focused on managing the underlying condition. The prognosis of systemic amyloidosis is typically poor. The severity of organ involvement, especially cardiac, is the most important prognostic factor.[9] Prog-nosis of a single organ or localized amyloidosis is good and may be treated symptomatically or by surgical intervention when there is a functional or esthetic deficit.

LIPOID PROTEINOSIS
Description

Lipoid proteinosis (LP) is a rare genodermatosis also known as hyalinosis cutis et mucosae or Urbach-Wiethe disease. It is caused by loss of function mutations in the *ECM1* gene that results in the deposition of an amorphous hyaline material in the skin and mucosal membranes. LP is more common in areas where consanguineous mar-riages take place.[10]

Clinical Features

Disease onset is usually in early infancy or, rarely, after a few years. Hoarseness is often the first sign and one of the most striking clinical manifesta-tions.[11] A pathognomonic sign for LP is the pres-ence of multiple firm, beaded papules along the eyelid margins, termed *moniliform blepharosis*.[12]

Accumulation of amorphous material may result in nodular, diffusely enlarged, and thickened labial and buccal mucosa (**Fig. 2**), and tongue. The pa-tient may develop waxy yellow-white submucosal plaques and nodules, thickening of the sublingual frenum and epiglottis, and gingival enlargement (**Fig. 3**A). The oropharyngeal mucosa may seem pale, and indurated resulting in restriction of mouth opening and tongue movement, and difficulty in swallowing.[10] The tongue may become firm and have a "wooden hard" consistency.[10] Ductal ste-nosis may cause recurrent salivary gland swelling.

Most patients, in the early disease, present with recurrent blistering and subsequent acneiform scarring, predominantly on the face and extrem-ities. Over time, the lesions may vary from waxy yellow papules and nodules to hyperkeratotic pla-ques in areas exposed to mechanical friction, to generalized skin thickening (**Fig. 3**B). Scalp involvement may lead to scarred alopecia. Bilat-eral intracranial calcifications develop in the late stage of the disease.[11] Seizures are, thus, an important neurologic sequela.[13] Other neurologic manifestations include social and behavioral changes, memory deficits, and mental retardation.

Histopathology

A tissue biopsy of the affected site will show depo-sition of an acellular, eosinophilic hyaline material in the connective tissue, largely around the blood vessels, nerves, sweat glands, and hair follicles. This material is diastase-resistant and stains with periodic acid-Schiff (PAS).

Differential Diagnosis

LP may have overlapping clinical-histopathological features with systemic

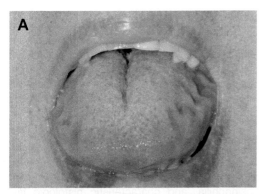

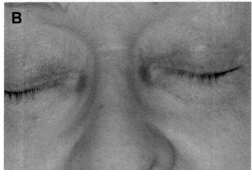

Fig. 1. Amyloidosis. (*A*) Macroglossia with characteristic crenations along lateral borders of tongue, and (*B*) purpura in the periorbital region. (*Courtesy of* Susan Muller, DMD, Decatur, GA; with permission.)

amyloidosis, plasminogen deficiency, and erythropoietic protoporphyria. Amyloidosis and plasminogen deficiency can be excluded with Congo-red and Fraser-Lendrum stains, respectively.

Erythropoietic protoporphyria usually does not cause similar oral lesions.[14] The skin lesions may resemble dermatologic conditions like xanthomas and lesions of leprosy.[10,12]

Diagnosis and Management

Diagnosis is confirmed by histopathological findings on biopsy of mucosal and skin lesions. The presence of comma or bean-shaped intracranial calcifications in the temporal lobes or hippocampi is the most common radiographic finding.[11] In addition, genetic testing for the *ECM1* gene can confirm the disease. There is no evidence-based treatment of LP and the disease runs a stable, chronic course. Surgical excision or debulking of the mucosal lesions, especially of the laryngeal mucosa to avoid breathing difficulty, may be required in some cases. A tracheostomy may be necessary for improving the airway. Gingivectomy is effective for facilitating oral hygiene. Oral application of dimethyl sulfoxide,[15] acitretin,[11] and corticosteroids[16] has been reported to improve the symptoms but the efficacy of these treatments remains controversial. Most patients with LP have a normal life expectancy.

PYOSTOMATITIS VEGETANS
Description

Pyostomatitis vegetans (PV) is a rare inflammatory disorder that is considered an oral manifestation of inflammatory bowel disease (IBD). The most common association of PV is with ulcerative colitis and is often described as a specific marker of the

Fig. 2. Lipoid proteinosis. Bilateral submucosal nodules of the labial and buccal mucosa. (*Courtesy of* Brad Neville, DMD, Charleston, SC; with permission.)

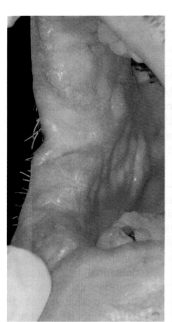
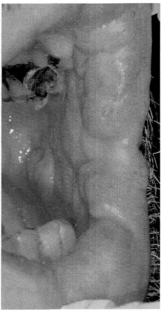

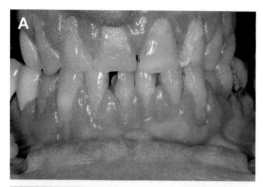

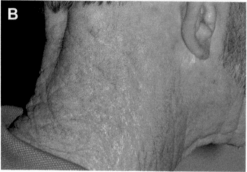

Fig. 3. Lipoid proteinosis. (*A*) Gingival hyperplasia due to infiltration of hyaline material, and (*B*) waxy papules on the back of neck. (*Courtesy of* Brad Neville, DMD, Charleston, SC; with permission.)

disease.[17,18] PV exhibits a male predilection and is most common in young and middle-aged adults.[17]

Clinical Features

Oral lesions may precede or appear with intestinal symptoms. Patients exhibit multiple slightly elevated, serpentine yellowish pustules on an erythematous base (**Fig. 4**).[17] The pustules rupture to form widespread shallow ulcerations resembling "snail track" ulcers. Rarely, tiny nodular lesions and hemorrhagic crusting may also be present.[19] As lesions progress they develop verrucous folds.[18] Any area of the oral mucosa may be affected, although the most commonly affected sites are the buccal and labial mucosa, hard and soft palate (**Fig. 5**), and gingiva.[18] Tongue and floor of the mouth are the least affected areas.[18,20] Most patients complain of mild tenderness or discomfort. The severity of PV may coincide with exacerbation of the underlying gastrointestinal disease.[21]

Histopathology

PV is usually characterized by the presence of intraepithelial and subepithelial eosinophilic abscesses. Marked edema may cause an acantholytic appearance of the involved epithelium.[8]

Differential Diagnosis

The differential diagnosis includes ulcerative and blistering conditions, such as pemphigus vulgaris, bullous pemphigoid, dermatitis herpetiformis, herpes simplex infections, syphilis, erythema multiforme, epidermolysis bullosa acquisita, bullous drug reaction, and Behçet disease.[18,20]

Diagnosis and Management

Diagnosis of PV is based on the combination of clinical features, association with IBD, peripheral eosinophilia, and characteristic histologic findings.[20] Identification of PV should facilitate investigation for IBD. The mainstay of management is primarily to treat the underlying gastrointestinal disease which usually results in the improvement of oral and skin lesions. Diet modulations, the use of corticosteroids, antispasmodic agents, and psychotherapy are the commonly used therapies. Oral lesions can be managed with local therapy such as topical corticosteroids. In the past, severe and recalcitrant lesions were treated with systemic corticosteroids,[17,21] dapsone,[17] and sulfasalazine.[18] More recently, newer disease-altering drugs, such as tumor necrosis factor-alpha (TNF-α) blockers, have been used to treat moderate to severe ulcerative colitis.[22] Janus kinase (JAK) inhibitors, such as tofacitinib (Xeljanz) and upadacitinib (Rinvoq), are used in cases where TNF blockers do not work well or are not tolerated.[23]

CROHN'S DISEASE
Description

CD is an inflammatory disorder of the gastrointestinal tract (GIT) that has oral and intestinal manifestations. Lesions can involve any part of GIT but predominantly affect the terminal ileum and colon.[24] The underlying etiology likely involves an inappropriate mucosal inflammatory response to intestinal bacteria.[25] CD has a bimodal age distribution, the first peak is seen in early adulthood and the second at 50 to 70 years of age.[25]

Clinical Features

The disease is characterized by periods of exacerbation and remission. The most common systemic manifestations include abdominal pain and prolonged diarrhea associated with rectal blood loss, fever, perianal fissure, arthralgia, and weight loss. Extraintestinal manifestations may affect the skin, eyes, and joints.[25] Oral manifestations are reported in approximately 0.5% to 37% of cases and may precede systemic manifestations.[26] Intraoral findings include

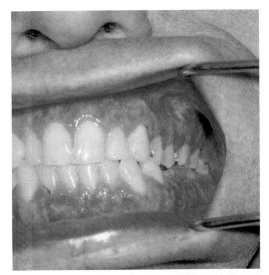

Fig. 4. Pyostomatitis vegetans. Characteristic yellowish-white linear serpentine pustules on the gingiva. (*From* Islam NM, Bhattacharyya I, Cohen DM. Common oral manifestations of systemic disease. Otolaryngol Clin North Am. 2011;44(1):161-182; with permission.)

mucogingivitis (linear ulcerations in the vestibule), gingival erythema (**Fig. 6**), diffuse persistent swelling of labial and buccal mucosa, cobblestone appearance of the mucosa (**Fig. 7**), soft tissue tags in the mucobuccal fold, and nodules in the vestibular retromolar area.[24] Nonspecific manifestations include angular cheilitis, glossitis, and aphthous ulcers.

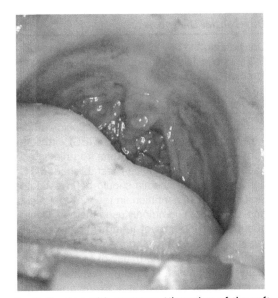

Fig. 5. Pyostomatitis vegetans. Ulceration of the soft palate and uvula in a 27-year-old woman.

Histopathology

Histologic findings involve the presence of non-caseating granulomas, composed of epitheliod histiocytes and lymphocytes, within the connective tissue. The presence of "skip lesions" in intestinal biopsy remains the first-line diagnostic tool in CD.[24]

Differential Diagnosis

Conditions that present with non-caseating granulomas, such as sarcoidosis, Wegener's granulomatosis, orofacial granulomatosis, and foreign body reaction should be considered in the differential diagnosis. Based on the clinical presentation of the cobblestoned oral mucosa, neurofibromatosis, multiple endocrine neoplasia (MEN) 2B, Cowden disease, Heck's disease, LP, and amyloidosis should be ruled out.[25]

Diagnosis and Management

Diagnosis is based on clinical assessment, physical examination, gastrointestinal endoscopy, laboratory, and histologic examination.[24] Oral lesions typically resolve once systemic corticosteroid therapy is initiated to suppress the abnormal inflammatory process. Topical steroids may be beneficial in providing symptomatic relief. Biological agents such as infliximab, tocilizumab, and adalimumab are reported to be effective in managing CD in those who cannot tolerate or are refractory to standard therapy.[24,25] Exclusion diet is beneficial in some patients. Maintenance of remission can be achieved with mercaptopurine.[27] Patients with CD are at risk of developing adenocarcinoma of the small intestine.[25] Therefore, periodic colonoscopy is a crucial aspect of management.

DIABETES MELLITUS
Description

Diabetes is a group of metabolic disorders that manifests as abnormally high glucose levels in the blood. Most oral manifestations of diabetes are evident in patients with poorly controlled disease.

Clinical Features

A strong relationship exists between diabetes and periodontal disease, to the extent that periodontal treatment can improve glycemic control.[28,29] Periodontal disease is more common and severe in patients who have poorly controlled diabetes than those with well-controlled disease or those without diabetes (**Fig. 8**).[30] Xerostomia has been reported in approximately one-third of patients.[31]

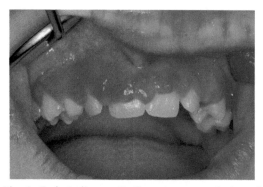

Fig. 6. Crohn's disease. Erythematous spongiotic and hyperplastic gingival lesions in a 12-year-old girl.

Diabetic patients are more susceptible to fungal infections, such as candidiasis, due to the reduced salivary flow and poor metabolic control. Mucormycosis may develop in poorly controlled type 1 diabetics with ketoacidosis. Taste dysfunction, burning mouth, delayed wound healing, and increased incidence of dental caries are more common in those with poorly controlled disease. An irreversible, nontender bilateral enlargement of parotid glands, called diabetic sialadenosis, may be seen in diabetic patients.[31]

Diagnosis and Management

Diagnosis is based on levels of fasting blood glucose and glycated hemoglobin (HbA1C), and glucose tolerance testing. Improved glycemic control can have a direct effect on periodontal health. Severe periodontal disease may be an indicator of disease progression.[32] Health care practitioners should, therefore, encourage regular dental evaluation for diabetic patients. Oral fungal

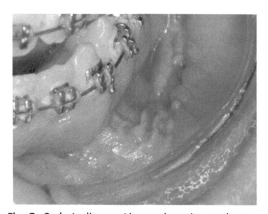

Fig. 7. Crohn's disease. Linear ulceration and corrugated, cobblestone appearance of the buccal mucosa and depth of the vestibule in a 14-year-old boy. (*Courtesy of* Kristin McNamara, DMD, Columbus, OH; with permission.)

infections should be treated with appropriate antifungal therapy.

IRON-DEFICIENCY ANEMIA
Description

Iron deficiency anemia is a common global health problem and the leading cause of anemia worldwide. It is commonly seen in young children, women of childbearing age, and elderly patients with chronic kidney disease.[33] Iron-deficiency anemia develops under four conditions: (1) Increased demand for red blood cells, particularly during childhood growth spurts and pregnancy; (2) Chronic blood loss, that may be associated with excessive menstrual flow or gastrointestinal disease such as peptic ulcers, diverticulosis; (3) Decreased intake of iron, especially in older adults; and (4) Decreased absorption of iron that can be seen in those with celiac sprue or complete gastrectomy.

Clinical Features

The condition is chronic and frequently asymptomatic, and thus may often remain undiagnosed. Systemic manifestations include weakness, fatigue, lightheadedness, palpitations, and shortness of breath, symptoms that are directly correlated to reduced oxygen supply to the body tissues. Oral signs and symptoms include atrophic glossitis, angular cheilitis, pale mucous membranes, erythema, tenderness, and burning sensation of the tongue (**Fig. 9**).[34] Alarmingly, children with iron-deficiency anemia tend to have a higher caries risk than the general population.[35]

Differential Diagnosis

Considering the oral signs and symptoms, vitamin B_{12} and folic acid deficiencies should be in the differential diagnosis.

Diagnosis and Management

Diagnosis is based on hematologic studies including complete blood count (CBC) with serum iron and ferritin levels, and total iron-binding capacity. Once the diagnosis is established, the underlying cause of anemia should be investigated. Oral iron supplementation, in the form of iron sulfate, is the most commonly used therapy. Usually, about 3 to 6 months of treatment is required to replenish iron stores and normalize the serum ferritin levels.[33] Long-term use of oral iron is associated with nausea, vomiting, constipation, and metallic taste. Intravenous iron therapy is more effective and increases hemoglobin levels more quickly than oral supplements, and may be given

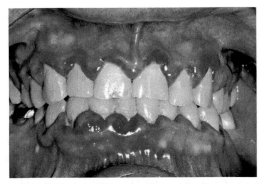

Fig. 8. Diabetes mellitus. Erythematous, hyperplastic gingival lesions in a patient with poorly controlled disease. (*From* Neville BW, Damm DD, Allen CM, Chi AC. Chapter 17: Oral Manifestations of Systemic Disease. Color Atlas of Oral and Maxillofacial Diseases. 1st ed. Elsevier; 2019; 505-528.)

to patients with severe anemia or malabsorption problems.[33]

PERNICIOUS ANEMIA
Description

Pernicious anemia (PA) is an autoimmune condition caused due to lack of vitamin B_{12} (cobalamin), either because of malabsorption or inadequate intake. PA is particularly common in elderly patients.[36] The condition is commonly caused by a lack of intrinsic factor (IF) which is produced by parietal cells of the stomach and needed for vitamin B_{12} absorption, thereby leading to impaired absorption of cobalamin.[8] This is common in those with autoimmune atrophic gastritis, and a possible role of *Helicobacter pylori* is postulated in its etiopathogenesis.[37] A reduced ability to absorb

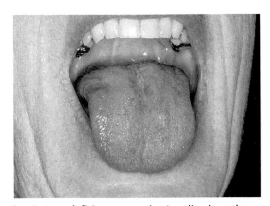

Fig. 9. Iron-deficiency anemia. Localized erythematous patches affecting the dorsal tongue. (*From* Islam NM, Bhattacharyya I, Cohen DM. Common oral manifestations of systemic disease. Otolaryngol Clin North Am. 2011;44(1):161-182; with permission.)

vitamin B_{12} may also develop in patients who have had gastric bypass surgery.[8] Because cobalamin is derived from animal sources, strict vegetarians may develop vitamin B_{12} deficiency.

Clinical Features

Like most anemias, nonspecific signs and symptoms include weakness, fatigue, headache, and shortness of breath. Vitamin B_{12} maintains myelin sheath throughout the nervous system; therefore, one of the most prominent manifestations of PA is neurologic impairment.[38] Patients may report tingling, or numbness of extremities, paresthesia, difficulty in walking, dementia, and irritability. Oral manifestations comprise atrophic glossitis or a bald tongue due to atrophy of papillae on the dorsal tongue, diffuse or focal patchy areas of mucosal erythema (**Fig. 10**), painful tongue, stomatitis, and burning sensation of the oral mucosa.

Differential Diagnosis

Patients with nutritional deficiencies of folic acid, iron, riboflavin, and niacin may exhibit similar symptoms and these should be considered in the differential diagnosis. Both vitamin B_{12} deficiency and folic acid deficiency cause megaloblastic anemia, and it is important to distinguish between the two conditions. Treatment of PA with folic acid will resolve the anemia and oral symptoms, but reduced myelin production will cause progressive damage to the central nervous system.

Diagnosis and Management

Diagnosis is based on CBC, estimation of serum vitamin B_{12} levels, and gastric biopsy if blood and bone marrow results are normal.[39] Detection of serum antibodies to IF is highly specific for PA.[38] The Schilling test that highlights the abnormal absorption of cobalamin has become obsolete. However, the Schilling test and IF antibody detection remain the gold standard for the diagnosis of PA.[36]

Early diagnosis and intervention are essential for treatment to be effective because the reversibility of neurologic symptoms relies predominantly on this.[39] Treatment typically consists of intramuscular injections of vitamin B_{12} at regular intervals, with a maintenance dose once every 2 months in the presence of and every 3 months in the absence of neurologic symptoms.[38] Oral cobalamin therapy is not preferred for patients with severe symptoms but may be used for long-term maintenance treatment.[38] Patients with autoimmune gastritis are predisposed to gastric carcinoma.[40] It is thus, extremely important to regularly screen such patients.

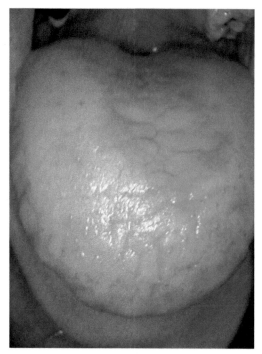

Fig. 10. Pernicious anemia. Glossitis exhibiting a red, smooth appearance, and focal red patches on the central portion of the dorsal tongue in a 56-year-old woman.

SCURVY
Description

Scurvy results from a nutritional deficiency of ascorbic acid or vitamin C. Lack of ascorbic acid affects the hydroxylation of amino acids proline and lysine resulting in suppression of collagen synthesis, the main organic component of many tissues including dentin, bone, and gingiva. Today, the incidence of scurvy is rare, especially in developed countries. Groups at risk include people with poor nutritional health and those dependent on others for care, including elderly persons living alone, alcoholics, drug addicts, and those with psychological or developmental problems.

Clinical Features

The disease has a slow onset. Nonspecific symptoms in the early stage, approximately 3 to 6 months after dietary intake falls below 10 mg/d, include fatigue, weakness, general lethargy, loss of appetite, irritability, myalgias, and arthralgias. Classic manifestations that appear sometime later comprise bleeding abnormalities due to the fragility of capillary walls. These lesions range from purpura, petechiae, ecchymoses, epistaxis, perifollicular and subperiosteal hemorrhage, and hemarthrosis, to bleeding gums.

Oral lesions are characterized by swollen and hyperplastic gingiva that may appear smooth, bluish-red, soft, friable, and bleed spontaneously on minor trauma (**Fig. 11**). Lesions usually start in the interdental areas. Severe vitamin C deficiency can lead to "scorbutic gingivitis," which is characterized by ulcerative gingivitis with periodontal pocket development and tooth loss.[41] Studies suggest that a local irritant like dental calculus can directly precipitate an inflammatory reaction.[42]

Other cutaneous manifestations include hyperkeratotic lesions, poor wound healing, corkscrew hair, nail changes, and alopecia.[43] Subperiosteal hemorrhages can result in intense bone pain and the inability to walk. As ascorbic acid performs an important function in the immune system and absorption of iron, its deficiency may lead to a higher incidence of infections and anemia, respectively.

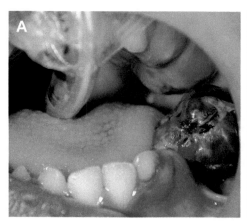
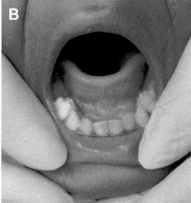

Fig. 11. Scurvy. (*A*) Severe gingival swelling and hyperplasia with hematoma formation, and (*B*) Complete resolution following 10 days of vitamin C supplementation. (*Courtesy of* Tina Woods, DMD, Charleston, SC)

Differential Diagnosis

The differential diagnosis of scurvy is broad and includes hematological abnormalities, vasculitis, drug-induced gingival hyperplasia, infection, vitamin D, K, and zinc deficiency, trauma to legs and joints (because of inability to walk), and leukemia. A thorough history and radiographs can eliminate trauma as an etiology. CBC and coagulation studies can rule out hematological abnormalities, vitamin deficiency, and leukemia.

Diagnosis and Management

Confirmatory laboratory tests include the determination of serum ascorbic acid levels. Generally, a vitamin C level of less than 0.1 mg/dL is confirmatory.[44] A positive capillary fragility test is an almost common finding.[44] Vitamin C supplementation is the only effective therapy. The recommended daily allowance of vitamin C is 45 mg/d for children and 60 mg/d for adults.[42] The prognosis for scurvy is excellent.

CLINICS CARE POINTS

- A multidisciplinary approach between physicians and dentists in the diagnosis and management of systemic conditions is of prime importance in achieving optimal clinical outcomes.

- Any unexplained changes in the oral mucosa that cannot be attributed to local trauma or other factors should be followed up in a timely manner. A biopsy should be performed for lesions that are persistent or recurrent, change physical characteristics, appear worrisome, or do not respond to therapy.

- Biopsies of oral ulcerations are sometimes non-specific. Since oral ulcers are seen in a multitude of diseases, investigation of their etiology often requires meticulous history taking and an extensive medical workup.

- Patients who exhibit oral symptoms as the first sign of a systemic condition should be referred to their primary care physician for a comprehensive evaluation and appropriate treatment.

DISCLOSURE

The authors have nothing to disclose.

REFERENCES

1. Schenkein HA, Papapanou PN, Genco R, et al. Mechanisms underlying the association between periodontitis and atherosclerotic disease. Periodontol 2000 2020;83(1):90–106.
2. Del Pinto R, Pietropaoli D, Munoz-Aguilera E, et al. Periodontitis and Hypertension: Is the Association Causal? High Blood Press Cardiovasc Prev 2020; 27(4):281–9.
3. Chapple IL, Genco R. Diabetes and periodontal diseases: consensus report of the Joint EFP/AAP Workshop on Periodontitis and Systemic Diseases. J Periodontol 2013;84(4 Suppl):S106–12.
4. Hazenberg BP. Amyloidosis: a clinical overview. Rheum Dis Clin North Am 2013;39(2):323–45.
5. Penner CR, Muller S. Head and neck amyloidosis: a clinicopathologic study of 15 cases. Oral Oncol 2006;42(4):421–9.
6. Elad S, Czerninski R, Fischman S, et al. Exceptional oral manifestations of amyloid light chain protein (AL) systemic amyloidosis. Amyloid 2010;17(1): 27–31.
7. Thompson LD, Derringer GA, Wenig BM. Amyloidosis of the larynx: a clinicopathologic study of 11 cases. Mod Pathol 2000;13(5):528–35.
8. Neville BW, Damm DD, Allen CM, et al. Oral manifestations of systemic diseases. In: Oral and maxillofacial pathology. 4th edition. St Louis (MO): Elsevier; 2016. p. 751–800.
9. Deng J, Chen Q, Ji P, et al. Oral amyloidosis: A strategy to differentiate systemic amyloidosis involving the oral cavity and localized amyloidosis. Oral Dis 2019;25(3):670–5.
10. Frenkel B, Vered M, Taicher S, et al. Lipoid proteinosis unveiled by oral mucosal lesions: a comprehensive analysis of 137 cases. Clin Oral Investig 2017; 21(7):2245–51.
11. Dertlioglu SB, Calik M, Cicek D. Demographic, clinical, and radiologic signs and treatment responses of lipoid proteinosis patients: a 10-case series from Sanliurfa. Int J Dermatol 2014;53(4):516–23.
12. Lee KC, Peters SM, Ko YCK, et al. Oral manifestations of lipoid proteinosis in a 10-year-old female: A case report and literature update. Oral Surg Oral Med Oral Pathol Oral Radiol 2018;126(4):e228–32.
13. Koen N, Fourie J, Terburg D, et al. Translational neuroscience of basolateral amygdala lesions: Studies of Urbach-Wiethe disease. J Neurosci Res 2016;94(6):504–12.
14. Deshpande P, Guledgud MV, Patil K, et al. Lipoid proteinosis: a rare encounter in dental office. Case Rep Dent 2015;2015:670369.
15. Ozkaya-Bayazit E, Ozarmagan G, Baykal C, et al. [Oral DMSO therapy in 3 patients with lipoidproteinosis. results of long-term therapy]. Hautarzt 1997; 48(7):477–81.
16. Zhang R, Liu Y, Xue Y, et al. Treatment of lipoid proteinosis due to the p.C220G mutation in ECM1, a major allele in Chinese patients. J Transl Med 2014;12:85.

17. Chan SW, Scully C, Prime SS, et al. Pyostomatitis vegetans: oral manifestation of ulcerative colitis. Oral Surg Oral Med Oral Pathol Dec 1991;72(6): 689–92.

18. Hegarty AM, Barrett AW, Scully C. Pyostomatitis vegetans. Clin Exp Dermatol 2004;29(1):1–7.

19. Pazheri F, Alkhouri N, Radhakrishnan K. Pyostomatitis vegetans as an oral manifestation of Crohn's disease in a pediatric patient. Inflamm Bowel Dis 2010; 16(12):2007.

20. Atarbashi-Moghadam S, Lotfi A, Atarbashi-Moghadam F. Pyostomatitis vegetans: a clue for diagnosis of silent crohn's disease. J Clin Diagn Res 2016;10(12):ZD12–3.

21. Ficarra G, Cicchi P, Amorosi A, et al. Oral Crohn's disease and pyostomatitis vegetans. an unusual association. Oral Surg Oral Med Oral Pathol 1993; 75(2):220–4.

22. Lv R, Qiao W, Wu Z, et al. Tumor necrosis factor alpha blocking agents as treatment for ulcerative colitis intolerant or refractory to conventional medical therapy: a meta-analysis. PLoS One 2014;9(1): e86692.

23. Fiorino G, D'Amico F, Italia A, et al. JAK inhibitors: Novel developments in management of ulcerative colitis. Best Pract Res Clin Gastroenterol 2018;32-33:89–93.

24. Alrashdan MS, Safadi RA. Crohn's disease initially presenting with oral manifestations and managed with ustekinumab: A case report. Spec Care Dentist 2021;41(5):634–8.

25. Woo VL. Oral Manifestations of crohn's disease: a case report and review of the literature. Case Rep Dent 2015;2015:830472.

26. Tan CX, Brand HS, de Boer NK, et al. Gastrointestinal diseases and their oro-dental manifestations: Part 1: Crohn's disease. Br Dent J 2016;221(12): 794–9.

27. Aguirre A, Nugent CA. Images in clinical medicine: oral manifestation of crohn's disease. N Engl J Med 2015;373(13):1250.

28. Grossi SG. Treatment of periodontal disease and control of diabetes: an assessment of the evidence and need for future research. Ann Periodontol 2001;6(1):138–45.

29. Darre L, Vergnes JN, Gourdy P, et al. Efficacy of periodontal treatment on glycaemic control in diabetic patients: a meta-analysis of interventional studies. Diabetes Metab 2008;34(5):497–506.

30. Moore PA, Weyant RJ, Mongelluzzo MB, et al. Type 1 diabetes mellitus and oral health: assessment of periodontal disease. J Periodontol 1999;70(4): 409–17.

31. Islam NM, Bhattacharyya I, Cohen DM. Common oral manifestations of systemic disease. Otolaryngol Clin North Am 2011;44(1):161–82, vi.

32. Thorstensson H, Kuylenstierna J, Hugoson A. Medical status and complications in relation to periodontal disease experience in insulin-dependent diabetics. J Clin Periodontol 1996;23(3 Pt 1): 194–202.

33. Camaschella C. Iron-deficiency anemia. N Engl J Med 2015;372(19):1832–43.

34. Wu YC, Wang YP, Chang JY, et al. Oral manifestations and blood profile in patients with iron deficiency anemia. J Formos Med Assoc 2014;113(2): 83–7.

35. Deane S, Schroth RJ, Sharma A, et al. Combined deficiencies of 25-hydroxyvitamin D and anemia in preschool children with severe early childhood caries: a case-control study. Paediatr Child Health 2018;23(3):e40–5.

36. Andres E, Serraj K. Optimal management of pernicious anemia. J Blood Med 2012;3:97–103.

37. Toh BH. Pathophysiology and laboratory diagnosis of pernicious anemia. Immunol Res 2017;65(1): 326–30.

38. Mohamed M, Thio J, Thomas RS, et al. Pernicious anaemia. BMJ 2020;369:m1319.

39. Goonewardene M, Shehata M, Hamad A. Anaemia in pregnancy. Best Pract Res Clin Obstet Gynaecol 2012;26(1):3–24.

40. Kuipers EJ. Pernicious anemia, atrophic gastritis, and the risk of cancer. Clin Gastroenterol Hepatol 2015;13(13):2290–2.

41. Nishida M, Grossi SG, Dunford RG, et al. Dietary vitamin C and the risk for periodontal disease. J Periodontol 2000;71(8):1215–23.

42. Fontana M. Vitamin C (ascorbic acid): clinical implications for oral health–a literature review. Compendium 1994;15(7):916–8, 920 passim; quiz 930.

43. Kitcharoensakkul M, Schulz CG, Kassel R, et al. Scurvy revealed by difficulty walking: three cases in young children. J Clin Rheumatol 2014;20(4): 224–8.

44. Halligan TJ, Russell NG, Dunn WJ, et al. Identification and treatment of scurvy: a case report. Oral Surg Oral Med Oral Pathol Oral Radiol Endod 2005;100(6):688–92.

Reactive and Nonreactive White Lesions of the Oral Mucosa

Sarah G. Fitzpatrick, DDS

KEYWORDS

- Oral cavity • White lesions • Leukoplakia • Developmental • Reactive • Premalignant • Malignant

KEY POINTS

- Developmental oral white lesions are often bilateral/symmetric, slow changing, and present for a long duration.
- Reactive oral white lesions frequently present along areas of chronic trauma such as occlusal plane of the buccal mucosa/tongue or edentulous alveolar ridge crest and often appear shaggy, without distinct demarcation.
- Idiopathic oral white lesions may overlap with reactive/premalignant lesions and may require additional follow-up to confirm diagnosis.
- Verrucous carcinoma may be mistaken for a nonmalignant lesion even on biopsy due to benign histologic appearance or sampling issues.

INTRODUCTION

White lesions of the oral mucosa demonstrate a full spectrum of etiologies including developmental, reactive, immune-related, idiopathic, and premalignant or malignant conditions. Developmental lesions develop early or later on in life, are often present bilaterally or symmetrically, and are generally stable over time. Reactive lesions may have an obvious traumatic source or be more nuanced in presentation. Immune-related white lesions, most commonly oral lichen planus or oral lichenoid mucositis, may fluctuate in clinical presentation and severity and even remit.

Lichenoid conditions are covered extensively in Chapter 4 and thus will only be discussed in this article in the context of differential diagnosis. In addition, lesions related to immunosuppression such as oral hairy leukoplakia (OHL) may also be considered in a differential diagnosis of white lesions and are addressed in Chapter 3. White lesions of candidiasis are addressed in Chapter 1 and may also be considered in the differential diagnosis but can often be clinically distinguished from other entities as superficially adherent plaques that wipe off easily, although hyperplastic candidiasis may overlap more significantly with other plaque-like white lesions of the oral cavity.

Many white lesions with nonobvious traumatic etiology and an uncertain behavior may fit into a group of lesions termed idiopathic leukoplakia, hyperkeratosis-nonreactive, or keratosis of unknown significance (KUS). This group may also have significant overlap with early dysplastic lesions or lesions within the proliferative verrucous leukoplakia (PVL) spectrum. Premalignant lesions with unifocal or multifocal presentation may present as white lesions with varying levels of surface change and divergent clinical features, and malignant lesions such as verrucous carcinoma (VC) may present only as an isolated papillary white lesion resembling a large papilloma/condyloma.

Although some white lesions of the oral cavity may be diagnosed clinically, the extent of clinical

Conflict of Interest/Funding: The author discloses no commercial or financial conflicts of interest or any funding sources for this article.

Department of Oral and Maxillofacial Diagnostic Sciences, University of Florida College of Dentistry, PO Box 100414, Gainesville, FL 32610, USA

E-mail address: sfitzpatrick@dental.ufl.edu

Oral Maxillofacial Surg Clin N Am 35 (2023) 237–246
https://doi.org/10.1016/j.coms.2022.10.010

overlap between premalignant and benign oral white lesions may often necessitate a biopsy to accurately manage many of these conditions.

Developmental or Hereditary Lesions

Developmental oral lesions may be hereditary or acquired and commonly or rarely encountered. Two examples at differing ends of this spectrum are leukoedema, which occurs commonly with an imprecise etiology and white sponge nevus (WSN), a rare autosomal dominant condition.

Leukoedema represents one of the most common white lesions in the oral cavity and may represent a variation of normal anatomy.[1] Although the etiology is unknown, it is generally thought to be developmental in origin, and irritation may also play a role with some studies noting increased incidence in patients using tobacco or betel products.[2,3] Leukoedema is a common occurrence in patient populations with higher melanin pigmentation levels of the skin, occurring in up to nearly 90% of patients of African American ethnicity, for example, with incidence increasing among patients within a population as level of pigmentation in the skin increases.[1,2,4] It may occur in both children and adults. Leukoedema presents bilaterally in over 90% of cases.[4] The clinical presentation of leukoedema is striking and characteristic, with a diffuse homogenous milky white appearance to the buccal mucosa, sometimes with a wrinkled appearance, that disappears when the tissue is stretched out – a feature that differentiates it from all other white lesions (**Fig. 1**). Although the diagnosis rarely requires a biopsy, the histologic appearance exhibits hyperparakeratosis with marked intracellular edema without atypia or dysplasia, which may resemble other conditions such as WSN, OHL, or traumatic hyperkeratosis. Unlike lesions of OHL, no nuclear inclusions of Epstein–Barr virus are observed, and immunohistochemical testing using EBER (Epstein-Barr encoding region) in-situ hybridization would be expected to be negative.

WSN is an autosomal dominant condition with variable clinical expression associated with mutation of keratin 4 and 13 genes.[1,5] It generally presents at an early age suggesting hereditary origin and is most frequently bilateral in nature.[1] The buccal mucosa is most frequently affected but the tongue, labial mucosa, floor of mouth, or gingiva, or non-oral mucosal locations may also be involved.[6,7] Clinically, the lesions present as asymptomatic thick corrugated diffuse white plaques, which require differentiation from premalignant oral lesions (**Fig. 2**). Similar oral lesions accompanied by ocular lesions may be seen in *hereditary benign intraepithelial dyskeratosis* (*HBID*), though this condition has been typically identified in a fairly narrow ancestry profile originating in the eastern United States.[8,9] Other genodermatoses such as dyskeratosis congenita may also have overlapping clinical presentation but with a wider range of non-oral signs and symptoms.[6] Histologically, WSN demonstrates hyperparakeratosis and intracellular edema similar to leukoedema, but also exhibits intracellular degeneration of keratinocytes with eosinophilic deposits in a perinuclear manner that is distinctive to this condition. Lesions of HBID exhibit hyperparakeratosis with dyskeratosis and a "cell-within-a-cell" pattern without the perinuclear eosinophilic deposits noted in WSN.[8] WSN is asymptomatic and treatment is not necessary once the diagnosis has been established.

Reactive Lesions

Reactive lesions of the oral cavity are frequently white in appearance due to proliferation of the surface epithelium in response to chronic or acute trauma, often from chewing, aggressive toothbrushing, habitual cheek or tongue biting, or an irritation mediated contact reaction to a topical product such as chewing tobacco, cinnamon, gums/mints/lozenges, toothpastes, or mouth rinses. Traumatic hyperkeratosis clinically appears shaggy with poorly demarcated borders, often presents in a generalized or symmetric manner, and is frequently located in areas subjected to trauma such as the crest of the edentulous ridge or the occlusal plane of the buccal mucosa or lateral tongue.

Alveolar ridge hyperkeratosis (also known as benign alveolar ridge keratosis or BARK) is commonly found on edentulous ridges particularly in areas with opposing natural dentition. The retromolar pad is frequently affected in a bilateral manner (**Fig. 3**). Smokers are also commonly affected.[10,11] Lesions typically are limited to the crestal aspect of the alveolar ridge, often lack distinct borders, but may be symmetric and bilateral, particularly on the retromolar pad.[12] Ulceration or erythema should provoke concern for dysplasia or neoplasia. Histologic examination generally reveals hyperkeratosis with "wedge-shaped" hypergranulosis without dysplasia or atypia, sometimes with a surface corrugation that may overlap slightly with premalignant verrucous lesions such as those within the PVL spectrum.[10–12]

Frictional keratosis limited to the facial attached gingiva has rarely been described related most frequently to aggressive toothbrushing habit.[13] It may clinically and histologically overlap with PVL

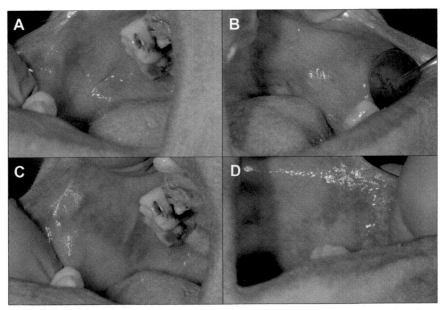

Fig. 1. Leukoedema exhibited by white milky lesions on right (*A*) and left (*B*) buccal mucosa that disappears when stretched out (*C, D*). (*Courtesy of* Hardeep Chehal, DDS, Omaha, NE.)

lesions due to sharp demarcation and thickened surface features. However, the location at the crest of the ridge and not the marginal gingiva is helpful in distinguishing it from PVL, and the histologic features are most similar to those of alveolar ridge hyperkeratosis. Also, no clinical progression is reported, and lesions resolve quickly after oral hygiene habits are altered.

Morsicatio buccarum and morsicatio linguarum (cheek chewing and tongue chewing, respectively) are parafunctional sequelae that patients may or may not be cognizant of as habits. Lesions generally appear as shaggy, poorly demarcated white lesions running along the occlusal plane of the buccal mucosa or tongue and are often symmetric in appearance (**Figs. 4** and **5**). The histologic

appearance exhibits hyperparakeratosis with frayed surface keratin, sometimes demonstrating adherent bacterial colonization, a lack of atypia or dysplasia, and minimal inflammation of the underlying connective tissue.[14]

More localized or asymmetric *traumatic/reactive hyperkeratosis,* such as those associated with a sharp or broken tooth or restoration, are often confined only to the area approximating the offending tooth, although lesions that do not resolve after adjustment or restoration of the tooth require biopsy to rule out dysplasia or neoplasia (**Fig. 6**). The histologic appearance of localized traumatic hyperkeratosis is characterized by hyperparakeratosis and acanthosis in most cases, without atypia or dysplasia.[14]

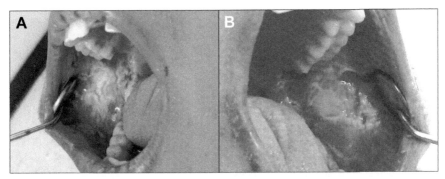

Fig. 2. White sponge nevus in an 18-year-old male patient exhibiting thick white lesions on right (*A*) and left (*B*) buccal mucosa. (*From* Belknap AN, Bhattacharyya I, Islam MN, Cohen DM. White sponge nevus, a rare but important entity. Oral 2021;1:307-312.)

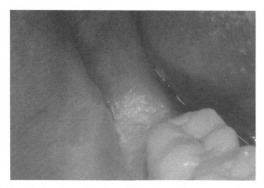

Fig. 3. Benign alveolar ridge hyperkeratosis of the retromolar pad. (*Courtesy* of Donald M. Cohen, DMD, MS, MBA; Indraneel Bhattacharyya, DDS, MSD; and Nadim M. Islam, DDS, BDS, Gainesville, FL.)

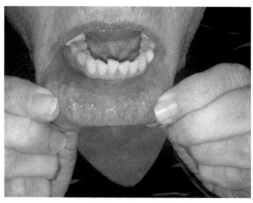

Fig. 5. Reactive hyperkeratosis secondary to lip chewing. (*Courtesy* of Donald M. Cohen, DMD, MS, MBA; Indraneel Bhattacharyya, DDS, MSD; and Nadim M. Islam, DDS, BDS, Gainesville, FL.)

Contact irritation stomatitis often appears as superficial sloughing or peeling adherent white plaques. Toothpaste ingredients such as sodium lauryl sulfate, triclosan, or tetrasodium pyrophosphate, along with various mouth rinses have been associated with superficial sloughing of the epithelium. It contains stringy or ropey exfoliating parakeratin or cellular debris that often can be noted in the vestibular areas but also may be widespread (**Fig. 7**).[14,15] Mild sensitivity may be present, or the lesions may be asymptomatic. Cessation of the offending agent generally resolves the condition. Other contact-related keratotic type lesions may appear thicker and more adherent, complicating the differential diagnosis. These have been associated with chronic use of cinnamon, gums/mints/lozenges, or other products (**Figs. 8 and 9**). Amalgam restorations can also provoke a keratotic contact reaction in addition to a lichenoid appearing lesion.[14] If lesions cannot be resolved by discontinuation of a suspected agent, then a biopsy may be indicated. The histology of irritation contact hyperkeratotic lesions generally appears nonspecific and exhibits hyperkeratosis along with mucositis in some cases.[14]

Tobacco pouch keratosis is a distinct and separate entity with overlap between both reactive and potentially preneoplastic lesions. Most tobacco pouch keratoses are reversible, resolving if the habit is discontinued, suggesting a reactive etiology. The reaction may be secondary to nicotine itself, contaminants, flavoring agents, or other additives in the product.[15] However, lesions that do not resolve with tobacco cessation may exhibit atypia, dysplasia, or carcinoma, necessitating biopsy. Tobacco pouch keratosis is typically localized to the area of tobacco placement generally the mandibular or maxillary vestibule. It appears as a diffuse, wrinkled, or corrugated white surface change which blends into the surrounding areas (**Fig. 10**). Ulceration or erythema should provoke suspicion of dysplasia or neoplasia. Tobacco pouch keratosis

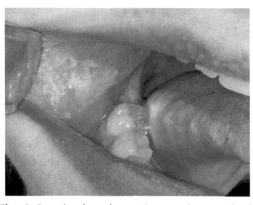

Fig. 4. Reactive hyperkeratosis secondary to cheek chewing (morsicatio buccarum) with biopsy compatible with severe hyperkeratosis. (*Courtesy of* Vishtasb Broumand, DMD, MD, Phoenix, AZ.)

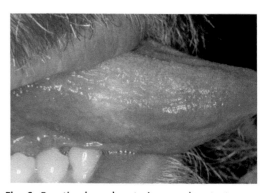

Fig. 6. Reactive hyperkeratosis secondary to trauma. (*Courtesy of* Alan Fetner, DMD, Jacksonville, FL.)

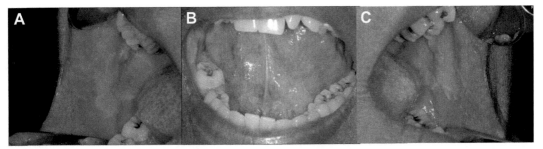

Fig. 7. Contact reaction to toothpaste and mouthwash exhibiting superficial sloughing and white lesions of the buccal mucosa and ventral tongue (*A–C*). (*Courtesy* of Donald M. Cohen, DMD, MS, MBA; Indraneel Bhattacharyya, DDS, MSD; and Nadim M. Islam, DDS, BDS, Gainesville, FL.)

exhibits hyperortho- or parakeratosis and acanthosis and may exhibit a wavy chevron-shaped keratotic surface.[14]

Idiopathic White Lesions/Lesions of Uncertain Behavior

White lesions in the oral cavity may also develop in the absence of obvious trauma, contact reaction, immune, or infectious etiology and also lack histologic features of dysplasia. Such lesions have been termed *idiopathic keratosis, keratosis of unknown significance, or hyperkeratosis-nonreactive*, and may represent a particularly difficult type of oral lesion to appropriately diagnose and manage. KUS lesions most frequently affect the lateral tongue, floor of mouth, and soft palate, all high-risk locations.[16] The lesions are sharply delineated and may show severe hyperkeratosis and mild atypia.[16] Although some of these lesions may be reactive, most represent early stages of dysplasia or PVL, early biopsies of which often demonstrate

severe hyperkeratosis but no overt dysplasia (**Fig. 11**).[16,17]

Findings from recent molecular analysis of KUS correlate well with those of mild epithelial dysplasia, emphasizing the need for close clinical follow-up and possible excision.[18,19]

Premalignant and Neoplastic Lesions

Leukoplakia is a clinical diagnosis defined as a white lesion without clearly obvious traumatic or infective etiology, and it is included in the category of oral potentially malignant disorders; however, it is accepted that a wide range of risk of malignant transformation exists within this spectrum and behavior may be uncertain.

Solitary leukoplakia may appear thin and homogenous and/or thicker with a verrucous or papillary surface. Leukoplakia with erythema (erythroleukoplakia) or ulceration is concerning for a higher risk of malignant transformation.[20] Leukoplakia with premalignant potential often exhibits a sharply

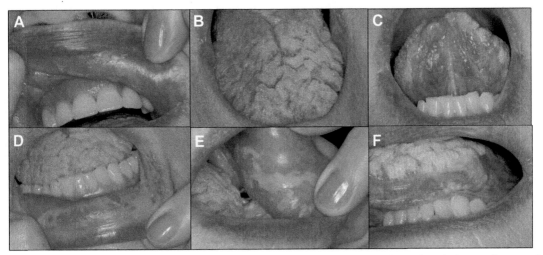

Fig. 8. (*A–F*) Reactive keratosis secondary to xylitol melt usage—patient with diffuse white lesions and usage of approximately 12 xylitol lozenges per day for symptoms of dry mouth. The patient was later diagnosed with Sjogren disease.

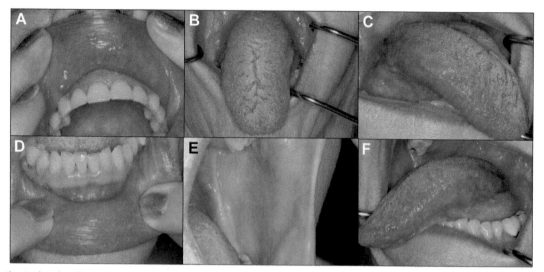

Fig. 9. (A–F): Full resolution of white lesions 2 weeks after discontinuation of xylitol lozenges. There were no recurrences of the lesions noted within 2 years of follow-up visits.

demarcated border, differentiating it from many reactive white lesions such as alveolar ridge keratosis. Solitary or localized leukoplakia is most common in men with tobacco use history and typically affects high-risk areas such as lateral/ventral tongue and floor of mouth. A malignant transformation rate of up to 22% is estimated for localized leukoplakia.[20] Risk factors that may increase the rate of malignant transformation include smoking status, high-risk location, nonhomogenous appearance, multifocal presentation, and large size.[21]

Early leukoplakic lesions may lack overt dysplasia.[20] Dysplastic lesions may include multiple abnormal architectural features such as

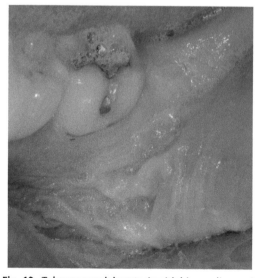

Fig. 10. Tobacco pouch keratosis with biopsy diagnosis of severe hyperkeratosis with acanthosis and mild atypia. (*Courtesy of* Jason Edwards, DMD, Tampa, FL.)

hyperkeratosis, with or without verrucous or papillary surface changes, sharply defined margins, multifocal or skip pattern, and epithelial proliferation.[22] Cytologically, the lesions may exhibit varying levels of epithelial dysplasia with increased nuclear size, mitoses, and individual cell keratinization.[22] A lichenoid response may be seen in response to these lesions and should not be diagnosed as oral lichen planus if dysplasia is present.[22] Treatment protocol generally depends on the level of dysplasia present and corresponding clinical factors.[23]

PVL, also termed *proliferative leukoplakia* if flat, presents clinically as a progressive, multifocal condition more frequently affecting older women, often with no history of tobacco use, which is an unusual risk profile for oral cancer. Unlike solitary leukoplakia, PVL favors the gingiva and buccal mucosa, but may occur in any oral location (**Fig. 12**). The lesions may clinically and histologically overlap with KUS or oral lichenoid mucositis, particularly in early stages, leading to diagnostic difficulty.[24] A hallmark feature of PVL is marginal linear gingival leukoplakia or "ring around the collar" (**Fig. 13**). This newly described pattern of markedly high-risk leukoplakia features progression of thick white lesions along the gingival margin of one or several teeth, often producing a circumferential ring of leukoplakia which is unlikely trauma-related.[25] A recent study indicated approximately 44% of PVL patients exhibited lichenoid clinical features, with a lower risk of malignant transformation noted in patients with early lichenoid presentation.[26] However, the presence of papillary or verrucous changes or dysplasia should exclude a diagnosis of oral lichen planus.[27]

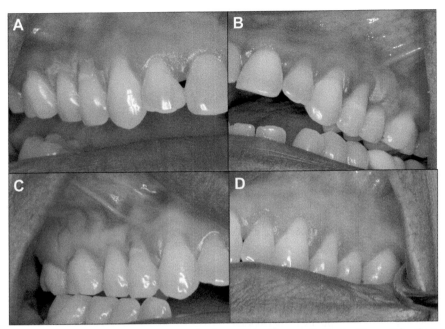

Fig. 11. Hyperkeratosis, nonreactive or keratosis of unknown significance. Patient with multifocal gingival white lesions with biopsy diagnosis consistent with verruco-papillary hyperkeratosis and lichenoid mucositis (*A, B*) and 3 years later full resolution of lesions without treatment intervention (*C, D*).

Histologically, many lesions of PVL exhibit marked architectural changes recognized as potentially premalignant such as verrucous, corrugated, or bulky keratosis but many lack outright dysplasia, complicating diagnosis.[28] Repeat biopsy over time in multiple locations is often necessary for diagnosis of PVL, and biopsy findings may range from simple hyperkeratosis, oral lichenoid mucositis, corrugated hyperkeratotic lesions absent dysplasia, bulky hyperkeratotic epithelial proliferations with or without dysplasia, and lesions suspicious for or with definitive features of VC or conventional squamous cell carcinoma (SCC).[24]

This condition is estimated to have a malignant transformation rate of between 50% and 100%, and progression of the malignant transformation is unpredictable in regards to time and location,

necessitating frequent follow-up and multiple biopsies.[29–32] Effective early intervention strategies are lacking for this condition, although patients with PVL who develop oral SCC have a better overall prognosis than those with traditional SCC as metastases less frequently result from PVL-associated SCC.[33,34]

VC may arise in late-stage PVL or as a solitary lesion. It is a rare subtype of oral SCC more common in men in non-PVL patients and has a predilection for the buccal mucosa, gingiva, and tongue.[22] It presents as a slow-growing predominantly white exophytic lesion with a thickened papillary or verrucous surface architecture (**Fig. 14**).

Verrucous hyperplasia as commonly seen in PVL is most likely a precursor to VC. These lesions

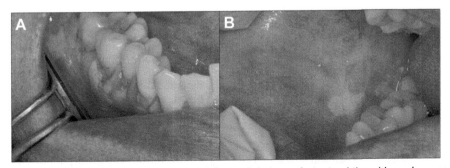

Fig. 12. Patient with proliferative verrucous leukoplakia with lesions of gingiva (*A*) and buccal mucosa (*B*).

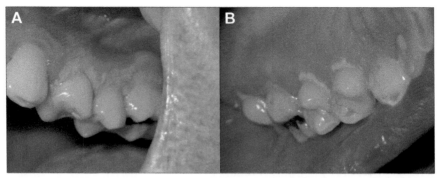

Fig. 13. Marginal linear gingival leukoplakia demonstrated by white lesions following the gingival margin exhibiting a collar-like pattern on both the buccal (*A*) and lingual (*B*) marginal gingiva. Biopsy was consistent with verruca-papillary hyperkeratosis with focal chronic lichenoid mucositis. (*Courtesy* of Donald M. Cohen, DMD, MS, MBA; Indraneel Bhattacharyya, DDS, MSD; and Nadim M. Islam, DDS, BDS, Gainesville, FL.)

lack definite evidence of invasion but demonstrate substantial epithelial proliferation causing diagnostic difficulty in some cases.[35] A variety of diagnostic terms such as *atypical verrucous proliferation/hyperplasia* have been used for especially proliferative examples of this lesion, but all should be viewed with high levels of suspicion for premalignant potential.[36,37]

VC presents with a markedly thickened, papillary, or verrucous surface epithelium with broad cohesive, pushing borders extending well into the underlying connective tissue and/or muscle. VC appears to be histologically benign due to the lack of separate individual invasive islands of tumor and a bland cytologic appearance. Features of dysplasia are usually absent, which also contributes to potential misdiagnosis. Pronounced keratin clefting is generally present and a reactive inflammatory response in the superficial connective tissue is frequent.[38] Adequate sampling on biopsy is imperative to achieving an accurate diagnosis. Verrucous carcinoma is associated with a more favorable prognosis than conventional oral SCC, but it may evolve into conventional oral SCC in 20% of cases.[22]

SUMMARY

White lesions within the oral cavity represent some of the most commonly encountered types of oral pathologic entities and may frequently cause diagnostic difficulty both clinically and histologically due to overlapping features between conditions. Consideration of both clinical history and appearance of the lesions is important in distinguishing benign from potentially malignant or malignant lesions. Warning signs include high-risk location, sharply demarcated borders, thickened, plaque-like, papillary, or verrucous lesions, erythroplakia, asymmetry, or the presence of isolated lesions with no apparent source of trauma, large or enlarging size, multiple recurrences, or a pattern of marginal linear gingival leukoplakia (ring around the collar) are all important and must be recognized to provide appropriate management.

CLINICS CARE POINTS

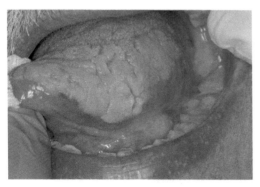

Fig. 14. Verrucous carcinoma exhibiting a thickened white proliferation on the dorsal and lateral tongue. (*Courtesy of* Indraneel Bhattacharyya, DDS, MSD.)

White lesions in high-risk locations require careful, long-term follow-up, including lesions on the floor of mouth, lateral and ventral tongue, the lingual frenum, marginal gingiva, tonsillar pillars, and lateral soft palate.

- Premalignant oral white lesions often exhibit distinctive clinical features such as unilateral/isolated location, larger size, sharp demarcation, verrucous/papillary surface, progressive growth, or distinctive growth patterns such as marginal linear gingival leukoplakia ("ring around the collar").

- Biopsies signed out as hyperkeratosis-nonreactive, or keratosis of unknown significance, correlate well with those of mild epithelial dysplasia, and require heightened surveillance or complete excision.

- Verrucous carcinoma may present as an isolated papillary white lesion resembling a large papilloma/condyloma.

REFERENCES

1. Pinna R, Cocco F, Campus G, et al. Genetic and developmental disorders of the oral mucosa: epidemiology; molecular mechanisms; diagnostic criteria; management. Periodontol 2000 2019;80:12–27.
2. Martin JL. Leukoedema: a review of the literature. J Am Med Assoc 1992;84(11):938–40.
3. Huang B-W, Lin C-W, Lee Y-P, et al. Differential diagnosis between leukoedema and white spongy nevus. J Dental Sci 2020;15:554–5.
4. Safadi RA, Shaweesh AI, Hamasha AA, et al. The significance of age group, gender and skin complexion in relation to the clinical distribution of developmental oral mucosal alterations in 5-13 year-old children. J Stomatol Oral Maxillofac Surg 2018;119:122–8.
5. Westin M, Rekabdar E, Blomstrand L, et al. Mutations in the genes for keratin-4 and keratin-13 in Swedish patients with white sponge nevus. J Oral Pathol Med 2018;47:152–7.
6. Bezerra KT, Leite TC, Roza ALOC, et al. White sponge nevus: a condition not always clinically suspected. J Cutan Pathol 2020;47:22–6.
7. Kurklu E, Ozturk S, Cassidy AJ, et al. Clinical features and molecular genetic analysis in a Turkish family with oral white sponge nevus. Med Oral Patol Oral Cir Bucal 2018;23(2):e144–50.
8. Jham BC, Mesquita RA, Aguiar MCF, et al. Hereditary benign intraepithelial dyskeratosis: a new case? J Oral Pathol Med 2007;36:55–7.
9. Bui T, Young JW, Frausto RF, et al. Hereditary benign intraepithelial dyskeratosis: report of a case and re-examination of the evidence for locus heterogeneity. Opthalmic Genet 2016;37(1):76–80.
10. Almazyad A, Li C-C, Woo S-B. Benign alveolar ridge keratosis: clinical and histopathologic analysis of 167 cases. Head Neck Pathol 2020;14:915–22.
11. Bellato L, Martinelli-Klay CP, Martinelli CR, et al. Alveolar ridge keratosis – a retrospective clinico-pathological study. Head Face Med 2013;9:12.
12. Natarajan E, Woo S-B. Benign alveolar ridge keratosis (oral lichen simplex chronicus): a distinct clinicopathologic entity. J Am Acad Dermatol 2008;58(1):151–7.
13. Mignogna MD, Fortuna G, Leuci S, et al. Frictional keratosis on the facial attached gingiva are rare clinical findings and do not belong to the category of leukoplakia. J Oral Maxillofac Surg 2011;69:1367–74.
14. Muller S. Frictional keratosis, contact keratosis and smokeless tobacco keratosis: features of reactive white lesions of the oral mucosa. Head Neck Pathol 2019;13:16–24.
15. Wang W, Woo S-B. Histopathologic spectrum of intraoral irritant and contact hypersensitivity reactions: a series of 12 cases. Head Neck Pathol 2021;15:1172–84.
16. Woo S-B, Grammer RL, Lerman MA. Keratosis of unknown significance and leukoplakia: a preliminary study. Oral Surg Oral Med Oral Pathol Oral Radiol 2014;118:713–24.
17. Alabdulaaly L, Almazyad A, Woo S-B. Gingival leukoplakia: hyperkeratosis with epithelial atrophy is a frequent histopathologic finding. Head Neck Pathol 2021;15:1235–45.
18. Villa A, Hanna GJ, Kacew A, et al. Oral keratosis of unknown significance shares genomic overlap with oral dysplasia. Oral Dis 2019;25:1707–14.
19. Stojanov IJ, Woo S-B. Malignant transformation rate of non-reactive oral hyperkeratosis suggests and early dysplastic phenotype. Head Neck Pathol 2022;16:36–374.
20. Woo S-B. Oral epithelial dysplasia and premalignancy. Head Neck Pathol 2019;13:423–39.
21. Kerr AR, Lodi G. Management of oral potentially malignant disorders. Oral Diseaes 2021;27:2008–25.
22. Muller S, Tilakaratne WM. Update from the 5th edition of the World Health Organization classification of head and neck tumors: tumours of the oral cavity and mobile tongue. Head Neck Pathol 2022;16:54–62.
23. Pentenero M, Sutera S, Lodi G, et al. Oral leukoplakia diagnosis and treatment in Europe and Australia: Oral Medicine practitioners' attitudes and practice. Oral Dis 2022. https://doi.org/10.1111/odi.14301.
24. Thompson LDR, Fitzpatrick SG, Muller S, et al. Proliferative verrucous leukoplakia: an expert consensus guideline for standardized assessment and reporting. Head Neck Pathol 2021;15:572–87.
25. Upadhyaya JD, Fitzpatrick SG, Islam MN, et al. Marginal linear gingival leukoplakia progressing to "ring around the collar" – an ominous sign of proliferative verrucous leukoplakia. J Periodontol 2021;92:273–85.
26. Barba-Montero C, Lorenzo-Pouso AI, Gandara-Vila P, et al. Lichenoid areas may arise in early stages of proliferative verrucous leukoplakia: a long-term study of 34 patients. J Oral Pathol Med 2022;1–9.
27. Cheng Y-SL, Gould A, Kurago Z, et al. Diagnosis of oral lichen planus: a position paper of the American

Academy of Oral and Maxillofacial Pathology. Oral Surg Oral Med Oral Pathol Oral Radiol 2016;122: 332–54.

28. Odell E, Kujan O, Warnakulasuriya S, et al. Oral epithelial dysplasia: recognition, grading and clinical significance. Oral Dis 2021;27:1947–76.

29. Gonzales-Moles MA, Warnakulasurya S, Ramos-Garcia P. Prognosis parameters of oral carcinomas developed in proliferative verrucous leukoplakia: a systematic review and meta-analysis. Cancers 2021;13:4843.

30. Alkan U, Bachar G, Nachalon Y, et al. Proliferative verrucous leukoplakia: a clinicopathological comparative study. Int J Oral Maxillofac Surg 2022. Epub ahead of print June 2022.

31. Ibanez de Mendoza IL, Lorenzo Pouso AI, Aguirre Urizar JM, et al. Malignant development of proliferative verrucous/multifocal leukoplakia: a critical systematic review, meta-analysis and proprosal of diagnostic criteria. J Oral Pathol Med 2022;51:30–8.

32. Palaia G, Bellisario A, Pampena R, et al. Oral proliferative verrucous leukoplakia: progression to malignancy and clinical implications. Systematic review and meta-analysis. Cancers 2021;13:4085.

33. Pereira Faustino IS, de Pauli Paglioni M, Linhares de Almeida Mariz BA, et al. Prognostic outcomes of oral squamous cell carcinoma derived from proliferative verrucous leukoplakia: a systematic review. Oral Dis 2022. Epub ahead of print February 2022.

34. Borgna SC, Clarke PT, Schache AG, et al. Management of proliferative verrucous leukoplakia: justification for conservative approach. Head and Neck 2017;39:1997–2003.

35. Akrish S, Eskander-Hashoul L, Rachmiel A, et al. Clinicopathologic analysis of verrucous hyperplasia, verrucous carcinoma, and squamous cell carcinoma as part of the clinicopathologic spectrum of oral proliferative verrucous leukoplakia: a literature review and analysis. Pathol Res Pract 2019;215:152670.

36. Muller S. Oral epithelial dysplasia, atypical verrucous lesions, and oral potentially malignant disorders: focus on histopathology. Oral Surg Oral Med Oral Pathol Oral Radiol 2018;125:591–602.

37. Zain RB, Kallarakkhal TG, Ramanathan A, et al. Exophytic verrucous hyperplasia of the oral cavity – application of standardized creteria for diagnosis from a consensus report. Asian Pac J Cancer Prev 2016;17:4491–501.

38. Thompson LDR. Verrucous squamous cell carcinoma. Ear Nose Throat J 2021;100(5S): 540S–541S-S.

Acute Immune-Mediated Lesions of the Oral Cavity

Molly Housley Smith, DMD[a],*, Mark Mintline, DDS[b]

KEYWORDS

- Aphthous stomatitis • Behçet • Contact stomatitis • Erythema multiforme
- Granulomatosis with polyangiitis

KEY POINTS

- Acute immune-mediated lesions of the oral cavity (AIML) of the oral mucosa arise suddenly and often are self-limited. They may be associated with systemic, multisystem inflammatory disease.
- Thorough clinical examination with medical, dental, and family history is vital in the diagnosis and classification of many of these conditions.
- The oral health care provider plays a pivotal role in the management of AIML, especially because oral manifestations may be the presenting sign for underlying systemic disease.
- Although all AIML have the potential to be recurring and/or relapsing, recurrences of some AIML are preventable with early diagnosis and proper management.

APHTHOUS STOMATITIS
Recurrent Aphthous Stomatitis

Recurrent aphthous stomatitis (RAS) or canker sores is a disease of unknown cause characterized by recurrent painful ulcers of the unattached oral mucous membranes. The lesions typically begin in childhood or adolescence and are characterized as single or multiple round or ovoid ulcerations with inflammatory halos.[1] RAS is one of the most common diseases of the oral mucosa with a reported worldwide prevalence of 10% to 15%.[2] A single triggering agent has not been identified, and investigators theorize that an altered local immune response to a variety of factors may induce aphthae. Approximately 80% of individuals with RAS report his or her first ulceration before the age of 30 years.[3] Commonly reported predisposing factors include stress, trauma, allergies, nutritional deficiencies, genetic predisposition, and hematologic abnormalities. Patients with frequent recurrences should be evaluated for systemic disorders (**Table 1**) that result in identical-appearing ulcerations termed aphthous-like ulcerations.[4]

The three clinical variants of aphthous stomatitis (AS) are minor AS, major AS, and herpetiform AS. Minor AS, or Mikulicz aphthae, represent approximately 80% of patients with RAS and often begin in childhood.[3] Lesions present on nonkeratinized oral mucosa and are typically less than 1 cm in diameter (**Fig. 1**). Minor AS may be painful, but they heal spontaneously within 7 to 14 days without scarring. Major AS or Sutton disease occurs in approximately 10% of patients with RAS[3] and is characterized by ulcerations that are larger and deeper (**Fig. 2**). The onset of major AS is often after puberty. Major aphthae may take several weeks to heal and can result in mucosal scarring that can rarely lead to restricted mouth opening. Herpetiform AS occurs in approximately 10% of patients with RAS and demonstrates the greatest number of ulcerations and most frequent recurrences.[3] Herpetiform AS typically occurs during adulthood and is most common in women. Individual pinhead-sized (1 to 3 mm) ulcerations (**Fig. 3**) can coalesce into larger, irregular ulcerations (**Fig. 4**). The multiple small ulcerations resemble lesions associated with an intraoral herpes simplex infection, hence the

[a] Pathology and Cytology Laboratory, 290 Big Run Road, Lexington, KY 40503, USA; [b] WesternU Health Oral Pathology, 701 East 2nd Street, Room 3204, Pomona, CA 91766, USA
* Corresponding author.
E-mail address: molly.housley.smith@gmail.com

Oral Maxillofacial Surg Clin N Am 35 (2023) 247–259
https://doi.org/10.1016/j.coms.2022.10.007
1042-3699/23/© 2022 Elsevier Inc. All rights reserved.

Table 1 Systemic disorders associated with aphthous-like ulcerations	
Cause	**Example**
Rheumatic diseases	Behçet's disease Reactive arthritis Sweet's syndrome PFAPA syndrome MAGIC syndrome
Gastrointestinal diseases	Celiac disease Inflammatory bowel disease (ulcerative colitis; Crohn's disease)
Nutritional diseases	Iron; folate; zinc; B1; B2; B6; B12
Drug reaction	NSAIDs, beta-blockers
Immunocompromised states	HIV infection
Hematologic disorders	Cyclic neutropenia; leukemia

Abbreviations: HIV, Human immunodeficiency virus; MAGIC syndrome, mouth and genital ulcers with inflamed cartilage syndrome; NSAID, non-steroidal anti-inflammatory drug; PFAPA, periodic fever, aphthous stomatitis, pharyngitis, adenitis.

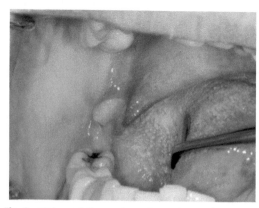

Fig. 2. Major aphthous ulceration: a large, deep ulceration of the pterygomandibular raphe was slow to heal and led to scarring (not pictured). (*Courtesy of* Mark Mintline, DDS, Pomona, CA.)

designation herpetiform AS; however, the etiology of herpetiform AS is unknown and unrelated to herpes simplex virus (HSV).

Aphthous ulcerations are typically diagnosed based on their clinical appearance and a suggestive patient history. Classically, RAS lesions are recurrent, small, and round ulcerations found on nonkeratinized oral mucosa that started during childhood. The histopathology of an aphthous ulceration is nonspecific, but a biopsy may rule out other clinical mimics. All three clinical variants of

AS may be further subdivided into simple and complex aphthosis to characterize healing and recurrence rates. In simple aphthosis, a few lesions are present, heal within 7 to 14 days, and rarely recur. In complex aphthosis, multiple lesions are present in a constant state of healing and development.

Effective treatment involves maintenance of the oral mucosal barrier, identification, and elimination of precipitating factors and minimizing recurrences. Most patients with mild aphthosis do not receive treatment, but ulcerations may be managed with over-the-counter anesthetics, medicaments, adhesive products, or topical corticosteroids. Ulcerations in major aphthosis are more resistant and often necessitate more potent topical corticosteroids, corticosteroid injections, or systemic corticosteroids. Patients with complex aphthosis should be evaluated to rule out possible triggers and underlying systemic disorders such

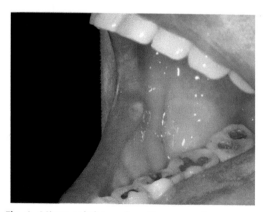

Fig. 1. Minor aphthous ulceration: a small, recurrent, and painful lesion of the labial mucosa. (*Courtesy of* Mark Mintline, DDS, Pomona, CA.)

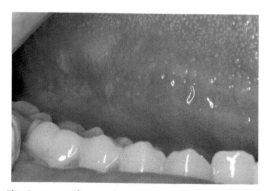

Fig. 3. Herpetiform aphthous ulcerations: a collection of pinhead lesions present on the lateral ventral tongue. (*Courtesy of* Molly Housley Smith, DMD, Lexington, KY.)

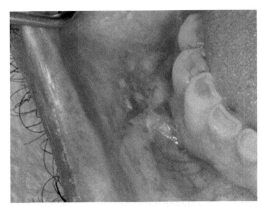

Fig. 4. Herpetiform aphthous stomatitis: multiple pinhead ulcerations of the labial vestibule coalesced into large and irregular areas of ulceration. (*Courtesy of* Mark Mintline, DDS, Pomona, CA.)

as cancer, infection, and other inflammatory or autoimmune conditions.

BEHÇET'S DISEASE

First described as a combination of oral and genital ulcerations (**Fig. 5**) and "hypopyon uveitis (**Fig. 6**),"[5] Behçet's disease (BD) is a rare, chronic, multisystem and relapsing inflammatory disorder of the vasculature classified as a "variable vessel vasculitis." Although the condition is chronic, the topic is discussed under this article because of the acute onset of oral ulcerations.

Owing to the increased historical prevalence of BD in individuals from the Mediterranean, Central Asia, and Far East regions, BD has been nicknamed "Silk Road Disease."[6] The disease affects between 1 in 1000 and 1 in 10,000 individuals, with Turkey having the highest incidence among

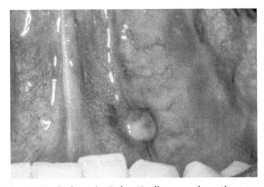

Fig. 5. Oral ulcers in Behçet's disease: ulcerations are identical to those found in aphthous stomatitis and often are small, painful, on unattached mucosa, and ovoid-to-round with an erythematous halo. (*Courtesy of* William T. Driebe, MD, and Eric Grieser, MD, Gainesville, FL.)

the endemic regions (20–420 per 100,000 people),[6,7] although other regions have seen an increase in cases due to immigration (especially to Germany, France, and the United States).[7] Interestingly, the ocular signs, pustular lesions, and vascular lesions are more often seen in men, and erythema nodosum and genital ulcerations are more frequently encountered in women.[6] In a large Iranian study analyzing 6,075 BD patients, 56% of patients were males, and 44% were females.[7]

Although the exact etiology and pathogenesis remain unclear, a variety of etiologic agents have been associated with BD, including microbial triggers/poor oral health,[8] immunological abnormalities, genetic factors, and endothelial dysfunction. Because familial cases of BD have been identified, many genetic links have been investigated, and a plethora of alleles have been implicated; HLA-B51, located on chromosome 6, is found most frequently in Japanese and Turkish patients with BD and is the best known HLA type associated with BD in general, affecting about 20% of patients.[6] Infectious agents, such as HSV 1, *Streptococcus sanguinis* (found in the oral microbiome), and others have been implicated.[6] Autoantibodies, particularly anti-endothelial cell antibodies as well as cytokines, also play important roles in this complex immune/environment interaction.

The signs and symptoms of BD are summarized in **Table 2**. Recurrent oral ulcerations are the presenting symptom in approximately 70% of BD patients,[9] and they are present in 86% to 100% of patients.[6] The oral ulcerations present identically to AS (see **Fig. 5**); thus, evaluation for other sites of involvement is critical to proper diagnosis. The ulcerations begin as painful papules that transform into round-to-ovoid ulcerations with erythematous halos and central white/yellow pseudomembranes. The ulcers predominantly affect the non-keratinized mucosa. Oral ulcerations do not appear to scar, whereas genital ulcerations are more commonly associated with scarring.[7]

There is no one laboratory test for BD, but rather, diagnostic criteria have been proposed. Two major classification systems for diagnosis are described: by the International Study Group for Behçet's disease (ISG) in 1990[10] and the International Criteria for Behçet's Disease (ICBD) in 2014.[11] In the ISG system, diagnosis is made on the presence of two of the following clinical signs/symptoms along with oral ulcerations: skin lesions, ocular involvement, genital ulcerations, and a pathergy test positivity. In the newest ICBD system, ocular involvement, genital ulcerations, and oral ulcerations are given two points each, whereas vascular involvement, skin lesions,

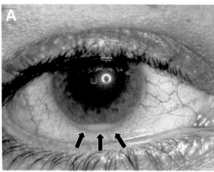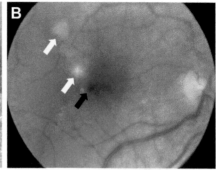

Fig. 6. Ocular manifestations of Behçet's disease: (*A*) inflamed conjunctival vasculature with inferior layered hypopyon (*arrows*) in the anterior chamber of the eye and (*B*) retinal photograph with vasculitis (*white arrow*) and retinitis (*black arrow*). (*Courtesy of* William T. Driebe, MD, and Eric Grieser, MD, Gainesville, FL.)

and neurologic signs/symptoms are each given one point. The patient is diagnosed with BD when the total number of points equates four or more.[11]

Patients with BD often are managed by a team of providers, which includes oral health care providers, rheumatologists, dermatologists, ophthalmologists, and gynecologists. Because poor oral health is associated with the etiology of BD, one simple step to help tame/manage oral ulcerations is regular dental checkups.[8] In order not to exacerbate the condition, it is not recommended that patients who have active oral ulcerations undergo dental treatment.[8] A variety of medications have been used to control the lesions, including topical and systemic corticosteroids, topical calcineurin inhibitors, anti-inflammatory agents, colchicine, azathioprine, mycophenolate mofetil, cyclosporine A, cyclophosphamide, thalidomide, methotrexate, lenalidomide, dapsone, pentoxifylline, interferon-α, anti-tumor necrosis factor (TNF)-α agents, anti-IL-1 and interleukin (IL)-6 agents.[6] Benzydamine hydrochloride mouth rinses have been used to decrease oral pain but not healing time.

Table 2	
Clinical signs and symptoms of Behçet's disease	
Site	**Clinical Manifestation**
Oral (86%–100%)	Painful papules, ulcerations, diffuse erythema of the soft palate/oropharynx
Genital (57%–93%)	Ulcerations most commonly on the scrotum in men and on the vulva for females
Skin	Extragenital aphthous ulcers; erythema nodosum-like lesions; papulopustular lesions; leukocytoclastic vasculitis
Ocular (40%–60%)	Bilateral panuveitis; anterior/posterior uveitis; conjunctivitis; recurrent attacks can lead to cataracts and glaucoma
Vascular	Superficial thrombophlebitis; deep vein thrombosis; arterial involvement (eg, arterial aneurysm, occlusion, stenosis of the aorta, femoral, or pulmonary vessels)
Cardiac	Endocarditis; pericarditis; valvular lesions; intracardiac thrombosis; myocarditis
Neurological (3%–25%)	Dural sinus thrombosis; aseptic meningitis; arterial vasculitis; meningoencephalitis; peripheral nerve involvement; psychiatric problems
Gastrointestinal (3%–26%)	Mucosal inflammation; ulcerations; diarrhea, abdominal pain, nausea
Musculoskeletal (45%–60%)	Arthritis; arthralgia; fibromyalgia; ankylosing spondylitis
Pulmonary	Vasculitis; fibrosis; infection; pleurisy; embolism

Data from Refs.[6,7]

Amlexanox and topical prostaglandin E2 gel also have been used to reduce ulcer size and pain as well as prevent the formation of new ulcers.[6] Topical steroids (eg, 0.05% fluocinonide gel, 0.05% augmented betamethasone dipropionate ointment, 0.5 mg/5 mL dexamethasone solution) have been used. Of note, oral phosphodiesterase-4 inhibitor apremilast (Otezla) is the first agent approved for use in treating BD in the United States.[12] Apremilast has been shown to reduce the pain and number of oral ulcerations, sustained over a period of 64 weeks of therapy.[12]

ALLERGIC CONTACT STOMATITIS

Contact stomatitis (CS) is characterized by inflammation and/or pain of the oral mucosa caused by exposure to an irritant or triggering allergen. Irritants include heat, trauma, and chemicals.[13] Irritants cause inflammation and activation of immunologic mediators without memory T-cells or antigen-specific immunoglobulins. Allergens associated with allergic CS (ACS) are numerous (**Box 1**), and the variable clinical appearance of ACS depends on the nature, potency, concentration, and period of exposure of the allergen.[14] Most ACS are delayed type hypersensitivity (Type IV) reactions and occur after an antigen exposure in a sensitized individual. Allergens that cause ACS may also contribute to exfoliative cheilitis and perioral dermatitis.[15]

CS is much less common than contact dermatitis and contact cheilitis, and the most affected sites for ACS are the buccal mucosa, gingiva, lateral borders of the tongue, and hard palate. Localized patterns of ACS are associated with focal allergens like dental restorations, orthodontic devices, or dental prostheses. Reactions from chewing gum and candies generally are also localized and most commonly affect the lateral border of the tongue and buccal mucosa. Generalized patterns are associated with foods, drinks, oral hygiene products, and flavoring agents.

The clinical features of acute ACS usually appear within hours of exposure to the allergen and can often be diagnosed with thorough history and examination. The most common symptom is a burning sensation, but itching and stinging are also reported. The appearance of the mucosa varies and may include erythema, swelling, vesicles (**Fig. 7**), erosions, and epithelial desquamation (**Fig. 8**). In mild cases, signs and symptoms typically resolve within 7 to 14 days after discontinuing or eliminating the allergen. In more advanced cases, antihistamines and anesthetics may be beneficial.

In chronic ACS, the oral epithelium is constantly or habitually exposed to an allergen. The oral mucosa can appear erythematous, white and hyperkeratotic (**Fig. 9**) or peel (see **Fig. 8**). In CS from artificial cinnamon flavoring, the lesions may mimic plasma cell gingivitis, morsicatio, oral hairy leukoplakia, or carcinoma.[16] Chronic or diffuse ACS or ACS may require extensive workups to discover the offending agent. The histopathology of ACS is nonspecific, but a biopsy may be required to rule out other conditions. Clinicians mainly review oral findings, rule out other etiologies, and correlate allergy skin test results to evaluate likely causes.[17] Direct testing of the oral mucosa may also be considered. A final diagnosis of ACS often is only rendered after the allergen has been removed, and recurrence of ACS following an antigen rechallenge confirms the diagnosis.

Box 1
Agents associated with oral contact stomatitis

- Oral hygiene products (toothpastes, mouth rinses)
- Foods (spices [eg, cinnamon], flavoring agents, chewing gum, candies)
- Gloves, rubber dams
- Dental restoration materials, orthodontic devices, acrylic denture materials, dental impression materials, gingival retraction cords, dental implants

Adapted from Feller L, Wood NH, Khammissa RA, Lemmer J. Review: allergic contact stomatitis. Oral Surg Oral Med Oral Pathol Oral Radiol. 2017;123(5):559-565.

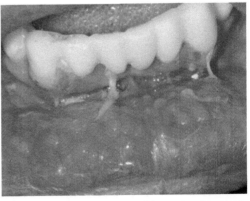

Fig. 7. Allergic contact stomatitis to aluminum chloride: superficial epithelial desquamation, erythema, and vesicles caused by the use of gingival retraction cord with aluminum chloride. (*Courtesy of* Mark Mintline, DDS, Pomona, CA.)

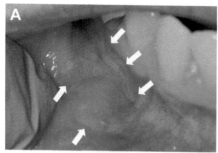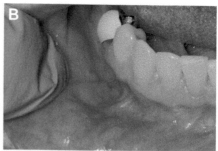

Fig. 8. Allergic contact stomatitis to mouth rinse: superficial desquamation (*white arrows*) in response to a mouthrinse (*A*) and resolution (*B*). (*Courtesy of* Molly Housley Smith, DMD, Lexington, KY.)

During investigations of suspected diffuse CS, patients should avoid mouthwash, mints, gum, products with cinnamon, and use toothpastes with flavoring agents or brush with baking soda. Patients should also forgo foods and beverages that can irritate the oral mucosa including carbonated, spicy, salty, and acidic aliments. The most important consideration for treatment of CS is identifying and avoiding the offending agent. When CS is due to a dental restoration or device, suitable replacements fabricated from different materials should be considered.[14]

ERYTHEMA MULTIFORME

Erythema multiforme (EM) is an acute, usually self-limited, cell-mediated immune reaction that often produces characteristic skin and mucosal lesions. It may be triggered by a wide variety of factors, including infections, medications, vaccines, or even systemic conditions or malignancies. Although EM used to be considered along the same pathologic spectrum as Stevens–Johnson Syndrome (SJS) and toxic epidermolysis necrolysis (TEN), recent evidence suggests that EM is a distinct disease process.[18,19]

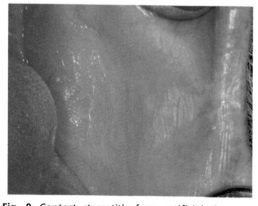

Fig. 9. Contact stomatitis from artificial cinnamon flavoring: patient reported a daily Atomic FireBall candy habit; lesion resolved 1 week after cessation. (*Courtesy of* Mark Mintline, DDS, Pomona, CA.)

EM affects a wide variety of individuals with no obvious sex or racial predilection. EM affects less than 1% of the population, predominantly adults younger than the age of 40 years[19]; however, a wide age range is noted.[20]

EM is initiated by a cell-mediated immune response, and most (greater than 90%) of the cases are correlated with infections, most notably herpes HSV type 1. The second most common trigger is *Mycoplasma pneumonia,* and there is a wide variety of infections that have been implicated in the etiology (**Table 3**).[19,21] Medications and vaccines are the initiating factor in anywhere from 10% to 50% of EM cases,[19,20,22] and autoimmune conditions such as irritable bowel disease and malignancies such as leukemias, lymphomas, gastric adenocarcinomas, and renal cell carcinoma also have been implicated.[19]

Patients with EM demonstrate skin and/or mucosal lesions that often begin on the skin as potentially burning or pruritic, red or pink papules that morph into plaques. By days 3 to 5, the lesions may take on a variety of clinical appearances. One of the most widely known and distinctive appearances for the condition is the "target" or "bull's eye" lesion (**Fig. 10**). In the beginning stages of the disease, the lesions are usually symmetrical, found on the extremities (**Fig. 11**), and may involve palms and soles.

Mucosal involvement is seen in 25% to 60% of patients with EM.[19] Most cases of mucosal involvement affect the oral cavity, although genital and ocular involvement may be present. Patients with mucosal lesions often also have prodromal symptoms, including malaise, fever, and weakness.[19,23] Intraoral lesions arise quickly and begin as red, edematous lesions which eventually erode or ulcerate, forming pseudomembranes (**Fig. 12**). Hemorrhagic crusting of the lips (**Fig. 13**) with significant intraoral ulcerations of the movable (nonattached) mucosal surfaces of the mouth is characteristic.[24] These lesions cause the patient

Table 3
Common triggers and associations with erythema multiforme

Infections	COVID-19 Cytomegalovirus Epstein–Barr virus Hepatitis B and C viruses Herpes simplex virus, types 1 and 2 Influenza virus *Mycoplasma pneumoniae* Vulvovaginal candidiasis
Vaccines	COVID-19 Hepatitis B Influenza Measles, mumps, rubella Meningococcal Smallpox

Medications	Antibiotics
	  Erythromycin
	  Nitrofurantoin
	  Penicillins
	  Sulfonamides
	  Tetracycline
	Antiepileptics
	Barbiturates
	Nonsteroidal anti-inflammatory drugs
	Phenothiazines
	Statins
	Sulfonamides
	Tumor necrosis factor-α inhibitors

Systemic conditions	Inflammatory bowel disease Malignancies (leukemia, lymphoma, renal cell carcinoma)

Adapted from Trayes, K. P., Love, G., & Studdiford, J. S. (2019). Erythema Multiforme: Recognition and Management. American family physician, 100(2), 82–88.

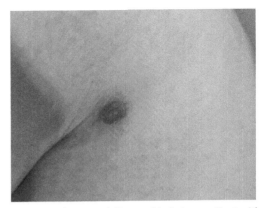

Fig. 10. Erythema multiforme skin lesion: patient with recurrent episodes of erythema multiforme presents with lesions on the leg, demonstrating a vague "targetoid" lesion with an outer erythematous ring. (*Courtesy of* Angela Tague, Sioux City, IA.)

significant pain and may impede the patient's ability to eat or take oral medications.

It is important to note that EM may recur. In one study of patients with recurrent EM, they had an average of six attacks per year.[19,25] In these cases, it is vital to carefully investigate for triggering infections or insulting medications.

EM is diagnosed clinically and does not require biopsy. Inquiring about the suddenness of disease onset, whether the patient started any new medications, and whether the patient recently was sick are vital questions in determining an accurate diagnosis. Once acute onset of the process has been established, one of the main differential diagnoses is primary herpetic gingivostomatitis (PHG), which also arises acutely, is self-limiting, is associated with fever and malaise, and can cause the

patient severe pain and inability to eat. Lack of or minimal attached mucosal involvement is the main useful clinical clue to help differentiate EM from PHG. When raised, papular target skin lesions are present or when the patient has a well-defined history of taking a new medication right before the outbreak, the clinical diagnosis is rather simple. Episodes of EM typically last from 2 to 5 weeks.[26] Both skin and mucosal lesions frequently heal without complications, although hyperpigmentation of the skin may be seen.[19,23]

With prominent skin involvement, another important differential diagnosis to rule out is SJS and TEN.[27]

In rare cases of persistent or longer lasting EM, biopsy may be useful in ruling out other chronic vesiculoerosive conditions (eg, erosive lichen planus, mucous membrane pemphigoid, and pemphigus vulgaris). The histopathologic features of EM show nonspecific ulceration with or without subepithelial separation, perivascular inflammation, and edema within the epithelial layer (**Fig. 14**).[24]

It is noteworthy that EM often is self-limiting, especially when cases are mild. Prophylactic antiviral therapy may be prescribed in cases when herpetic reactivation is suspected as the triggering agent.[19] Etiologic medications must be discontinued.

Because lesions are self-limiting, the use of corticosteroids is controversial.[24,28] Many patients, however, are treated with systemic and/or topical steroids with or without antihistamines. In cases with severe skin and mucosal involvement, the clinician may choose an agent that can work systemically and topically (eg, prednisolone taken in a "swish and swallow" fashion). Palliative care includes numbing agents and bland nutrient shakes to soothe the oral cavity while providing nutrition

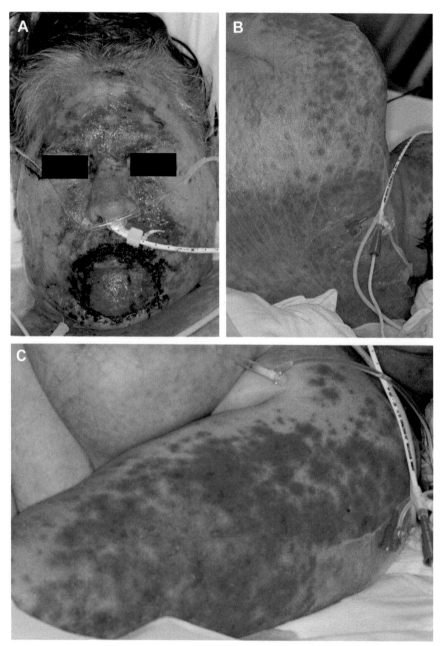

Fig. 11. Erythema multiforme skin lesions: patient presents with extensive skin and mucosal involvement (*A*), starting on the distal extremities and extending onto the back (*B*). Note that the stomach and chest appear to be spared of lesions (*C*). (*Courtesy of* Brent Newby, DDS, MD, Overland Park, KS.)

when solid food intake is nearly impossible due to severe pain. In severe involvement, patients may require hospitalization to administer intravenous (IV) fluids and replenish electrolytes.[19]

FIXED DRUG ERUPTIONS

Medications have long been associated with a variety of oral manifestations, many of which have

been or will be discussed further in other articles. Deserving of mention in this article, as it arises suddenly and can be confused with other entities within this article (namely EM), is the fixed drug eruption (FDE). An FDE is a lesion that occurs in the same location due to exposure to a specific medication.[29] Lesions can affect the skin, oral or genital mucosa.[24] Although FDE can present at any age, the most frequently affected individuals

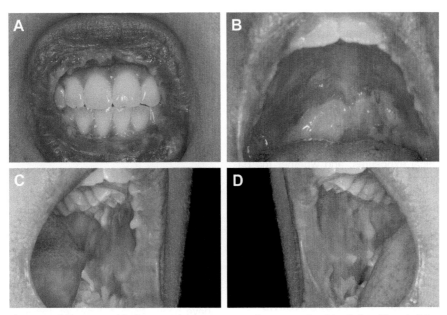

Fig. 12. Erythema multiforme oral lesions: patient present to the urgent health clinic with painful mouth ulcerations that affect the labial mucosa (*A*), soft palate (*B*), left (*C*), and right (*D*) buccal mucosa. Note that the hard palate and gingiva are spared. (*Courtesy of* Molly Housley Smith, DMD, Lexington, KY.)

are young-to-middle-aged adults. The median age ranges from 35 to 60 years.[30]

Over 100 medications have been implicated in the onset of FDE.[29] The medications that have been implicated in this process include acetaminophen, antihistamines, antiepileptics, nonsteroidal anti-inflammatory drugs, azole antifungals, antibiotic medications, and nicorandil.[24] Lesions begin within 24 hours of ingestion of the offending medication, and CD8+ T cells begin to move into the epidermis, producing pro-inflammatory factors that lead to epidermal necrosis.[30] The lesions are self-limited, likely because CD4+ regulatory

T cells subsequently produce anti-inflammatory cytokines which counteract the effect.[30] It also is noteworthy that specific HLA genes have been associated with FDE to specific medications.[30]

Although FDE occurs as an insult from offending medications, similar reactions may occur because of ingesting offending foods. These reactions have been termed "Fixed food eruptions" and can occur with a wide variety of foods, including strawberries, kiwis, cashew nuts, almonds, walnuts, seafood, and lentils. Food colorings (particularly yellow) also have been implicated.[30]

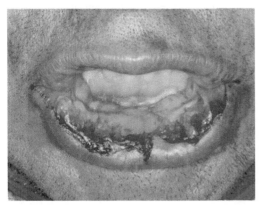

Fig. 13. Erythema multiforme lip lesions: Hemorrhagic crusting of the lower lip with ulcerations and erosions of the labial mucosa. (*Courtesy of* Mark Mintline, DDS, Pomona, CA.)

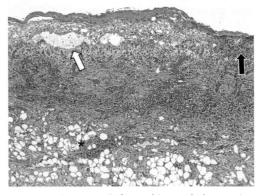

Fig. 14. Erythema multiforme histopathology: microscopic examination reveals vesicle formation (*white arrow*) with ulceration (*black arrow*), significant epithelial spongiosis, and deep perivascular inflammation (*asterisk*). (*Courtesy of* Molly Housley Smith, DMD, Lexington, KY.)

FDE of the oral cavity presents as bullae, ulcerations (**Fig. 15**), or erythematous areas. Patients may complain of a pain or burning sensation in the area. When on the skin, FDE manifest as a rash with or without overlying vesicles and/or bullae.[30] With each new time that the specific medication is ingested, additional sites may be affected.

Diagnosis of FDE is based on a thorough clinical examination and history (including list of medications, chemical exposures, and whether the patient has had before occurrence). Biopsy results are nonspecific and may demonstrate ulceration with perivascular inflammation. Therapy consists of finding and removing the offending medication.[24] If the patient and/or clinician are unsure about a particular medication or food, patch testing offers a safe method of evaluation.

GRANULOMATOSIS WITH POLYANGIITIS

First described as a separate entity by Friedrich Wegener in the 1930s,[31] granulomatosis with polyangiitis (GPA) is an immune-mediated necrotizing vasculitis of the small blood vessels. Notorious for being a painful and life-altering diagnosis, GPA can become fatal if not recognized rapidly and treated appropriately.[32] It characteristically affects the upper and lower respiratory tracts and the kidneys, whereas sometimes affecting the oral cavity. Because of the characteristic oral manifestations that may arise, oral providers are pivotal to early detection and management. This systemic condition is associated with circulating antineutrophil cytoplasmic antibodies (ANCA) directed against target antigens proteinase 3 (PR3) (75%) or myeloperoxidase (MPO) (20%), although a small percentage (5%) of patients demonstrate no known apparent association with any type of ANCA.[33,34]

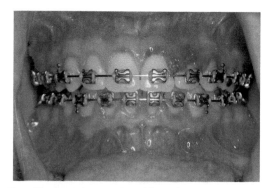
Fig. 16. Granulomatosis with polyangiitis: patient presents with red, pebbly, hyperplastic gingiva of the maxillary left facial gingiva. (*Courtesy of* Gary Altschuler, DMD, Gainesville, FL.)

GPA is rare; its prevalence has been estimated to be around 7 to -12 new cases per year per one million people.[35] Patients of all ages (8–99 years) have been affected; however, the average age at diagnosis ranges from 45 to 80 years.[31,33] Although GPA affects all races, Caucasians seem to be most affected.[31] Some investigators cite a slight male predominance for all ANCA-associated vasculitides;[33] however, a sex predilection is not apparently noted in GPA.[31]

Although some things are known about the pathogenesis of GPA, not as much is known about why it occurs; however, many associations have been made. GPA seems to be more common in the winter months. In addition, the presence of *Staphylococcus aureus* in the nasal mucosa has been associated with an increased incidence of relapse. A host of other factors have been implicated in GPA, including dust inhalation and exposure to silica.[35] Although rare, familial forms have been described.

GPA arises acutely over a period of several days or a period of a few months, and it may affect a

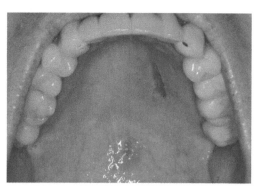
Fig. 15. Fixed drug eruption: patient presents with nonmigrating ulcerations of the hard and soft palate after taking the offending medication. (*Courtesy of* Molly Housley Smith, DMD, Lexington, KY.)

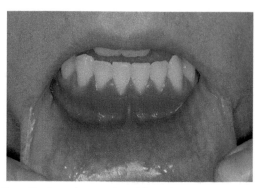
Fig. 17. Granulomatosis with polyangiitis: patient presents with fiery red facial gingiva. (*Courtesy of* Tina Woods, DMD, Charleston, SC.)

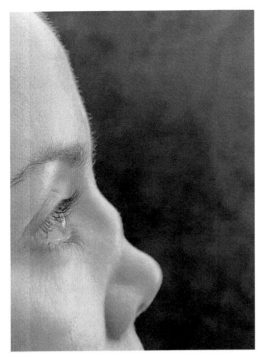

Fig. 18. Granulomatosis with polyangiitis: patient presents with characteristic "saddle nose" deformity in which the nasal bridge has collapsed. (*Courtesy of* Emily Kyne, Canada.)

limited area or a wide area of the body. The clinical manifestations depend on which areas of the body are affected. Of note, clinical involvement of the ear/nose/throat, lungs, and kidneys is referred to as "ELK." The disease process may begin with involvement of only one or two of the ELK areas, but can progress to the systemic form, especially when left untreated.[31] The upper respiratory tract is affected in 70% to 100% of cases, and the nasal cavity and paranasal sinuses are the sites most involved in the head and neck region (85%–100%). Critical for the oral provider, GPA can manifest as the characteristic "strawberry gingivitis" (**Fig. 16**) in which the patient's gingiva is red/purple in color (**Fig. 17**), hyperplastic, and demonstrates a bubbly or pebbled surface architecture. Another clinically evident feature is the presence of a "saddle nose" deformity in which the nasal bridge collapses due to necrosis of the vasculature in that area (**Fig. 18**).

The clinical indications for ANCA testing are numerous, but these indications include the presence of cutaneous/mucosal vasculitis with systemic features. Recommendations for how and when to test for GPA and other vasculitis disorders are outlined in the Revised 2017 International Consensus on Testing of ANCAs in Granulomatosis with Polyangiitis and Microscopic Polyangiitis.[36] High-quality antigen-specific assays for both PR3 and MPO are recommended as the primary screening method for those exhibiting oral lesions with evidence of necrotizing vasculitis.[36]

Biopsy specimens from the head and neck are often small and fragmented and may not be definitive, but they are useful to rule out other entities or to support a clinical diagnosis of GPA. Importantly, GPA may show subtle microscopic changes which only may be found by the pathologist under significant clinical suspicion, strengthening the notion that providing clinical details and descriptions aide the pathologist in making an accurate diagnosis.

Histopathologic examination of GPA often reveals oral mucosa that is densely inflamed with lymphocytes, plasma cells, macrophages, and/or multinucleated giant cells[32] (**Fig. 19**). Although rarer to find in oral biopsies, small vessel vasculitis and well-formed granulomas may be seen.[32] Collections of extravasated red blood cells often are seen, which correlate to the pebbly, erythematous appearance noted clinically.

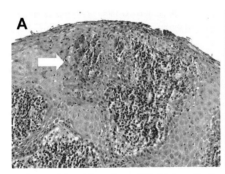
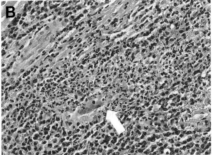

Fig. 19. Granulomatosis with polyangiitis histopathology: microscopic examination reveals dense inflammation with significant leukocytic exocytosis and accumulations of extravasated red blood cells (*A*). In the deeper stroma, small vessel walls are destroyed by significant inflammation (*white arrow*) (*B*). (*Courtesy of* Molly Housley Smith, DMD, Lexington, KY.)

Some vasculitides may be triggered by a variety of drugs, including propylthiouracil, minocycline, hydralazine, cocaine adulterated with levamisole, and antitumor necrosis factor agents.[33] Once the use of offending drugs has been excluded clinically, patients with GPA are treated with a plethora of immunosuppressive medications, including glucocorticosteroids, cyclophosphamide, rituximab, and mycophenolate mofetil.[33] A multidisciplinary approach with providers, including rheumatologists, oral clinicians, renal and respiratory physicians, otorhinolaryngologists, and ophthalmologists, is ideal to evaluate the extent of disease and treat the patient accordingly.

SUMMARY/DISCUSSION FOR WHOLE TOPIC

Some of the acute immune-mediated lesions of the oral cavity (AIML) are common and can be extremely painful, and a few are associated with systemic disease, which, if not caught early, can be detrimental to the patient's life. For all AIML, a thorough clinical history and evaluation with proper medical, dental, and family history are vital to early detection and therapy. The oral health care provider is an important member of the health care team for patients with these conditions, as oral manifestations may be the first sign of disease and knowledge of the oral microbiome, proper oral hygiene practices, and accurate oral examination technique are crucial to appropriate management of AIML.

CLINICS CARE POINTS

- Patients with recurrent oral ulcers must be quizzed as to the presence of genital, eye, and/or skin lesions to rule out Behçet's disease, erythema multiforme major, and granulomatosis with polyangiitis.

- When evaluating patients with erythema multiforme (EM), note that 90% are caused by infections and 10% to 50% by medications and vaccines.

- Oral EM resembles primary herpes but often recurs and rarely affects the attached gingiva.

- It is important to recognize patients with strawberry-like granular vascular lesions of the gingiva and evaluate for granulomatosis with polyangiitis, as it can become fatal if not recognized rapidly and treated appropriately

REFERENCES

1. Ship JA. Recurrent aphthous stomatitis. An update. Oral Surg Oral Med Oral Pathol Oral Radiol Endod 1996;81(2):141–7.
2. Lau CB, Smith GP. Recurrent aphthous stomatitis: A comprehensive review and recommendations on therapeutic options. Dermatol Ther 2022;35(6): e15500.
3. Belenguer-Guallar I, Jiménez-Soriano Y, Claramunt-Lozano A. Treatment of recurrent aphthous stomatitis. A literature review. J Clin Exp dentistry 2014; 6(2):e168–74.
4. Scully C. Clinical practice. Aphthous ulceration. N Engl J Med 2006;355(2):165–72.
5. Scherrer M, Rocha VB, Garcia LC. Behçet's disease: review with emphasis on dermatological aspects. Anais brasileiros de dermatologia 2017;92(4): 452–64.
6. Bulur I, Onder M. Behçet disease: New aspects. Clin Dermatol 2017;35(5):421–34.
7. Davatchi F, Chams-Davatchi C, Shams H, et al. Adult Behcet's disease in Iran: analysis of 6075 patients. Int J Rheum Dis 2016;19(1):95–103.
8. Mumcu G, Fortune F. Oral Health and Its Aetiological Role in Behçet's Disease. Front Med 2021;8:613419.
9. Park UC, Kim TW, Yu HG. Immunopathogenesis of ocular Behçet's disease. J Immunol Res 2014; 2014:653539.
10. Criteria for diagnosis of Behçet's disease. International Study Group for Behçet's Disease. Lancet (London, England) 1990;335(8697):1078–80.
11. International Team for the Revision of the International Criteria for Behçet's Disease (ITR-ICBD). The International Criteria for Behçet's Disease (ICBD): a collaborative study of 27 countries on the sensitivity and specificity of the new criteria. J Eur Acad Dermatol Venereol 2014;28(3):338–47.
12. Deeks ED. Apremilast: A Review in Oral Ulcers of Behçet's Disease. Drugs 2020;80(2):181–8.
13. Cifuentes M, Davari P, Rogers RS 3rd. Contact stomatitis. Clin Dermatol 2017;35(5):435–40.
14. Feller L, Wood NH, Khammissa RA, et al. Review: allergic contact stomatitis. Oral Surg Oral Med Oral Pathol Oral Radiol 2017;123(5):559–65.
15. Collet E, Jeudy G, Dalac S. Cheilitis, perioral dermatitis and contact allergy. Eur J Dermatol 2013;23(3): 303–7.
16. Müller S. Frictional Keratosis, Contact Keratosis and Smokeless Tobacco Keratosis: Features of Reactive White Lesions of the Oral Mucosa. Head neck Pathol 2019;13(1):16–24.
17. Tosti A, Piraccini BM, Peluso AM. Contact and irritant stomatitis. Semin Cutan Med Surg 1997;16(4): 314–9.
18. Lamoreux MR, Sternbach MR, Hsu WT. Erythema multiforme. Am Fam Physician 2006;74(11):1883–8.

19. Trayes KP, Love G, Studdiford JS. Erythema Multiforme: Recognition and Management. Am Fam Physician 2019;100(2):82–8.

20. Celentano A, Tovaru S, Yap T, et al. Oral erythema multiforme: trends and clinical findings of a large retrospective European case series. Oral Surg Oral Med Oral Pathol Oral Radiol 2015;120(6):707–16.

21. Jimenez-Cauhe J, Ortega-Quijano D, Carretero-Barrio, et al. Erythema multiforme-like eruption in patients with COVID-19 infection: clinical and histological findings. Clin Exp Dermatol 2020;45(7): 892–5.

22. Petruzzi M, Galleggiante S, Messina S, et al. Oral erythema multiforme after Pfizer-BioNTech COVID-19 vaccination: a report of four cases. BMC oral health 2022;22(1):90.

23. Sokumbi O, Wetter DA. Clinical features, diagnosis, and treatment of erythema multiforme: a review for the practicing dermatologist. Int J Dermatol 2012; 51(8):889–902.

24. Fitzpatrick SG, Cohen DM, Clark AN. Ulcerated Lesions of the Oral Mucosa: Clinical and Histologic Review. Head neck Pathol 2019;13(1):91–102.

25. Wetter DA, Davis M. Recurrent erythema multiforme: clinical characteristics, etiologic associations, and treatment in a series of 48 patients at Mayo Clinic, 2000 to 2007. J Am Acad Dermatol 2010;62(1): 45–53.

26. Heinze A, Tollefson M, Holland KE, et al. Characteristics of pediatric recurrent erythema multiforme. Pediatr Dermatol 2018;35(1):97–103.

27. Newkirk RE, Fomin DA, Braden MM. Erythema Multiforme Versus Stevens-Johnson Syndrome/Toxic Epidermal Necrolysis: Subtle Difference in Presentation, Major Difference in Management. Mil Med 2020;185(9–10):e1847–50.

28. Aurelian L, Ono F, Burnett J. Herpes simplex virus (HSV)-associated erythema multiforme (HAEM): a viral disease with an autoimmune component. Dermatol Online J 2003;9(1):1.

29. Patel S, John AM, Handler MZ, et al. Fixed Drug Eruptions: An Update, Emphasizing the Potentially Lethal Generalized Bullous Fixed Drug Eruption. Am J Clin Dermatol 2020;21(3):393–9.

30. Anderson HJ, Lee JB. A Review of Fixed Drug Eruption with a Special Focus on Generalized Bullous Fixed Drug Eruption. Medicina (Kaunas, Lithuania) 2021;57(9):925.

31. Greco A, Marinelli C, Fusconi M, et al. Clinic manifestations in granulomatosis with polyangiitis. Int J immunopathology Pharmacol 2016;29(2):151–9.

32. Geetha D, Jefferson JA. ANCA-Associated Vasculitis: Core Curriculum 2020. Am J kidney Dis : official J Natl Kidney Found 2020;75(1):124–37.

33. Jennette JC, Falk RJ, Bacon PA, et al. 2012 revised International Chapel Hill Consensus Conference Nomenclature of Vasculitides. Arthritis Rheum 2013;65(1):1–11.

34. Fonseca FP, Benites BM, Ferrari A, et al. Gingival granulomatosis with polyangiitis (Wegener's granulomatosis) as a primary manifestation of the disease. Aust dental J 2017;62(1):102–6.

35. Comarmond C, Cacoub P. Granulomatosis with polyangiitis (Wegener): clinical aspects and treatment. Autoimmun Rev 2014;13(11):1121–5.

36. Bossuyt X, Cohen Tervaert JW, Arimura Y, et al. Position paper: Revised 2017 international consensus on testing of ANCAs in granulomatosis with polyangiitis and microscopic polyangiitis. Nat Rev Rheumatol 2017;13(11):683–92.

Plasma Cell Gingivitis and Its Mimics

Rania H. Younis, BDS, MDS, PhD[a],*, Maria Georgaki, DDS, MSc, PhD[b],
Nikolaos G. Nikitakis, MD, DDS, PhD[b]

KEYWORDS

- Plasma cell gingivitis • Clinical features • Histologic features • Differential diagnosis • Treatment

KEY POINTS

- Plasma cell gingivitis is a distinct, benign inflammatory oral condition most often limited to the free and attached gingiva.
- Clinicopathologic correlation is required for diagnosis.
- The line of treatment depends on the severity of symptoms and esthetic concerns.
- Management can vary from identifying and eliminating the offending allergen to topical or systemic steroids.

PLASMA CELL GINGIVITIS

Plasma cell gingivitis (PCG) is a rare inflammatory oral condition characterized by a polyclonal proliferation of plasma cells in the subepithelial gingival tissue.[1] PCG is also known by a variety of other names such as atypical gingivostomatitis, plasmacytosis, idiopathic gingivostomatitis, and allergic gingivostomatitis.[2] Although etiopathogeneses remain unknown, several factors especially hypersensitivity to certain antigens (eg, toothpastes, oral rinses, chewing gums, spices) have been considered to play a crucial role.[3] However, most of these lesions are considered to be idiopathic.[2]

Clinical Features of Plasma Cell Gingivitis and Diagnostic Workup

PCG can affect any age and both genders with a higher prevalence in women. Clinically, it may involve any area of the mouth, with most cases presenting as lesions of rapid onset in the free and attached gingiva. Specifically, it can appear as localized or diffuse edematous, and erythematous gingival tissues which can easily bleed, lose its normal stippling, with or without surface ulcerations (**Fig. 1**). Usually, the lesions are asymptomatic but in some cases can cause pain[4] or even a burning sensation.[5] A characteristic of the disease is the absence of desquamation of the gingiva and a negative Nikolsky sign, which is helpful in differentiating it from other vesiculobullous diseases. White striations characteristic of lichenoid lesions is also usually absent. Other rare clinical presentations have been reported including those with a white keratotic component, papillomatous, cobblestone, nodular, or velvety appearance.[3] Diagnostic workup is based on the patient's history and clinicopathologic correlation, whereas a full blood count (leukemia), erythrocyte sedimentation rate (lupus, infection, inflammation), serum angiotensin converting enzyme (s-ACE) (sarcoidosis), antineutrophil cytoplasmic antibodies (granulomatosis with polyangiitis), and dermatologic patch testing for contact allergens[6,7] can be indicated to rule out the many mimics of PCG. Nonetheless, the diagnosis must be histologically confirmed.

Histopathologic Features of Plasma Cell Gingivitis

Microscopically, PCG consists of a dense plasma cell infiltrate in the subepithelial connective tissue

[a] Department of Oncology and Diagnostic Sciences, School of Dentistry, University of Maryland, 650 West Baltimore Street, 7th floor suite 7257, Baltimore, MD 21201, USA; [b] Department of Oral Medicine & Pathology and Hospital Dentistry, School of Dentistry, National and Kapodistrian University of Athens, 2 Thivon Street, 115 27, Goudi, Athens, Greece
* Corresponding author.
E-mail address: ryounis1@umaryland.edu

Oral Maxillofacial Surg Clin N Am 35 (2023) 261–270
https://doi.org/10.1016/j.coms.2022.10.003
1042-3699/23/© 2022 Elsevier Inc. All rights reserved.

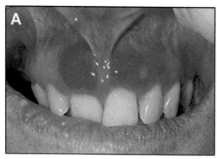
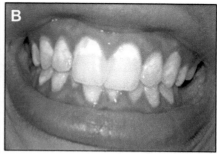

Fig. 1. Clinical presentations of plasma cell gingivitis. (A) Well-localized erythematous lesion of the anterior maxillary attached gingiva that extends to involve part of the alveolar mucosa, in a 63-year-old woman. (B) Diffuse erythematous lesion that involves the anterior maxillary and mandibular marginal gingiva and extends to the attached gingiva in some areas, in a 13-year-old patient with dental fluorosis. Patient proved allergic to Iodopropynyl butylcarbamate (IPBC), a preservative in personal care products. (Clinical Picture (B) Courtesy Dr Ronald S. Brown.)

(**Fig. 2**). Epithelium has been described as psoriasiform[6,8] and epithelial hyperplasia with elongated rete ridges, spongiosis, and loss of normal keratinization or papillary thinning and dyskeratosis can be also seen.[9] The stroma can be predominantly vascular. The histopathologic differential diagnosis includes monoclonal neoplastic processes like plasmacytoma, multiple myeloma (MM), Waldenström macroglobulinemia, and lymphoma[2,3,10] Immunohistochemistry and/or in situ hybridization of kappa (κ) and lambda (λ) immunoglobulin (Ig) light chains (**Fig. 3**), along with IgG, IgA, and IgM immunoglobulins,[4] should demonstrate the polyclonal origin of the plasma cell infiltrate to confirm the diagnosis of PCG. Special stains for infectious agents should be negative. The presence of large numbers of plasma cells also seen in chronic inflammatory periodontal diseases can sometimes cause difficulty in distinguishing ordinary gingival inflammation from PCG.[2] The presence of mixed inflammatory cells and the clinical correlation with the chronic nature of the periodontal disease can help distinguish it from PCG.[11]

Management of Plasma Cell Gingivitis

The management of PCG can be a challenge. There are no specific treatment protocols and management lacks international consensus about drug classes and regimens, often resulting in poor clinical outcome.[12,13] Generally, asymptomatic lesions may not require treatment; however, for symptomatic lesions or those causing esthetic concern, treatment is usually required. The clinician's first concern is to elicit from the patient's history possible exposure to allergens or causative factors (eg, chewing gums, certain food, cosmetics, and oral hygiene products).[7,10,14–16] If

temporal relation can be identified with the introduction of a specific agent, the lesions usually subside on removal of the causative factor. Although PCG does not respond to plaque control, attention should still be paid to local factors and mouthwash use, in order to reduce immunologic cell-mediated and cytokine-mediated responses that can complicate recovery. Treatment is usually symptom-based, with topical corticosteroids (0.05% clobetasol propionate, dexamethasone 0.5 mg/5 mL, fluocinonide 0.05%, triamcinolone acetonide 0.1%)[1,8] (**Fig. 4**). Response to antihistaminic chlorpheniramine maleate has been also reported.[17] For persistent cases, systemic steroids, immunomodulators, and sometimes antibiotics (doxycycline and 2% fusidic acid) have been elected.[1,4] PCG is generally an innocuous condition with no evidence of malignant transformation. Surgical excision and laser ablation have been reported to treat the condition, but the PCG lesions are usually recurrent if the causative factor was not identified or avoided.

CLINICAL DIFFERENTIAL DIAGNOSIS

The oral clinical differential diagnosis of the condition is very important as it can mimic a wide range of other entities such as medication-related gingival lesions, granulomatous lesions (foreign body gingivitis, sarcoidosis, and Crohn's disease), reactive lesions like spongiotic gingival hyperplasia, and less common, ligneous gingivitis.[9,12,18,19]

Medication-Related Gingival Lesions

Administration of several medications due to an underlying systemic disease can cause lesions similar to PCG. Chemotherapy can cause erythematous and ulcerative lesions of the oral cavity that can involve the gingiva.[20–22] Phenytoin,

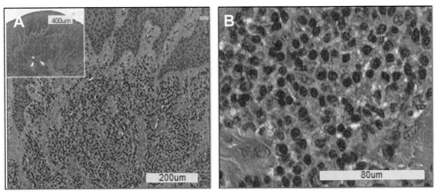

Fig. 2. Histopathologic features of plasma cell gingivitis. (*A*) H&E stain of soft tissue section demonstrating dense subepithelial inflammatory cell infiltrate divided by bundles of collagenous fibrous tissue. Inset of low power view shows intact overlying surface epithelium. (*B*) A higher power view of the inflammatory cell infiltrate in (*A*), demonstrating the predominant plasma cell component. The plasma cells present classic features of eccentric nucleus and abundant amphophilic cytoplasm. Some also demonstrating perinuclear eosinophilic halo (Russell bodies). The nuclei demonstrate cartwheel or clock-faced distribution of chromatin.

calcineurin inhibitors (cyclosporine), calcium-channel blockers (nifedipine, amlodipine, and oxodipine), and oral contraceptives are agents that most commonly cause drug-induced gingival enlargement.[23,24] These lesions usually manifest as firm enlargement of the gingiva. The swelling typically starts 1 to 4 months after drug administration in the interdental gingiva and progresses to involve the marginal and attached gingivae. The enlargement is usually diffuse and is more severe in the maxillary and mandibular anterior region. In some cases, the gingiva is edematous and erythematous and may mimic PCG. Histopathologically, the lesions consist of

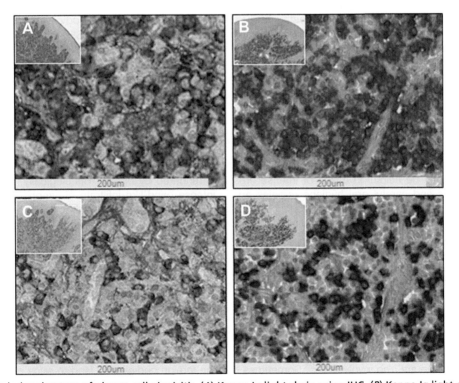

Fig. 3. Polyclonal nature of plasma cell gingivitis. (*A*) Kappa-Ig light chain using IHC. (*B*) Kappa-Ig light chain using ISH. (*C*) Lambda-Ig light chain using IHC. (*D*) Lambda-Ig light chain using ISH. IHC, immunohistochemistry; ISH, in situ hybridization.

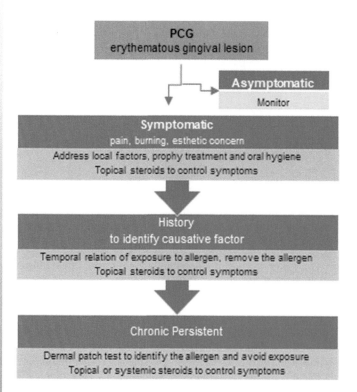

PCG
erythematous gingival lesion

Asymptomatic
Monitor

Symptomatic
pain, burning, esthetic concern
Address local factors, prophy treatment and oral hygiene
Topical steroids to control symptoms

History
to identify causative factor
Temporal relation of exposure to allergen, remove the allergen
Topical steroids to control symptoms

Chronic Persistent
Dermal patch test to identify the allergen and avoid exposure
Topical or systemic steroids to control symptoms

Fig. 4. Outline for clinical management of plasma cell gingivitis. Treatment directed identifying the causative factor and addressing symptoms.

epithelial hyperplasia, long rete ridges, hyperplastic fibrous and collagenous connective tissue, and chronic inflammation that lack the predominant plasma cell component of PCG. Diagnosis is based on the patient's history, clinical examination, and the bulky fibrous overgrowth that is usually easily identified as medication-induced gingival hyperplasia not PCG. The putative drug should be withdrawn if this is possible by the treating physician, as discontinuation of the drug leads to inhibition of the progression of the disease and even regression of the gingival hyperplasia. Gingivectomy may be helpful in cases of intense enlargements and careful oral hygiene remains an important parameter.[24]

Foreign Body Gingivitis

Foreign body gingivitis is a chronic inflammatory disease involving the marginal and/or attached gingiva and is due to the immune-mediated reaction against embedded foreign body material.[25] Clinically, the disease appears as solitary or multiple red or red and white lesions, sometimes resembling erosions, and frequently the interdental papillae are also involved.[25,26] Sometimes, the patients complain about pain and swelling of the gingiva. The clinical appearance may mimic desquamative gingivitis and lichen planus, and

only 50% of cases demonstrate granulomatous inflammation.[25] Foreign body gingivitis develops more often in women (68%–84%) with a mean age of 48 year old.[25,27] Most of the times, the development of the lesions is preceded by microtrauma from dental restoration or prophylaxis.[25,26] Factors that have been associated with the development of foreign body gingivitis include amalgam, dental crown placement, dental prophylaxis, orthodontic treatment, and periodontal surgery.[25] The lesions are often misdiagnosed as lichen planus or lichenoid reactions.[25] Diagnosis is rendered by biopsy. Histologically, there is an intense band-like infiltrate of lymphocytes at the submucosal-epithelial interface and keratinocyte degeneration. In the connective tissue, microdeposits of foreign body particles can be discerned in histiocytes and multinucleated giant cells.[25] The diagnostic criteria include the identification of foreign bodies in the connective tissue, where there is chronic inflammation and the presence of foreign bodies in at least two sequential tissue sections.[25] The most common detected element is silica in 94% of cases.[28] Silica is an ingredient of polishing paste and iatrogenic implantation of the foreign bodies may lead to silica granulomas. The second most frequent element is silicon followed by aluminum and titanium.[26] Foreign body gingivitis is not correlated to plaque and calculus accumulation, and hygiene measures targeting plaque prevention have no effect. Furthermore, in contrast to oral lichen planus, steroid therapy shows no clinical improvement.[25,27] Surgical excision and gingival grafting are nowadays controversial and mostly applied in extreme cases.[25] It is recommended to avoid air abrasion polishing in cases of the disease as further exacerbation is possible. Finishing and polishing of dental restorations close to soft tissues should be carried out carefully and in cases of gingival ulcerations or recent oral soft-tissue trauma, such dental treatment should be postponed after healing of the tissues.[26]

Orofacial Granulomatosis

Orofacial granulomatosis is a term used to describe the occurrence of granulomas in the orofacial region in the absence of any recognized systemic condition. Typically, orofacial granulomatosis presents as recurrent, persistent labial swellings, which result in enlargement of the lips. This condition may also be associated with oral ulceration, painless gingival overgrowth, and a cobblestone appearance of the buccal mucosa. Gingival manifestations are infrequently described in the literature and develop in 21% to 26% of patients.[19] Gingival involvement presents as gingival enlargement, that is usually red in color, smooth and shiny, with loss of stippling.[29] It can be either full-width or localized gingivitis. Biopsy is mandatory to establish diagnosis. Histopathologic examination reveals noncaseating granulomatous lesions and edema. Periodic Acid–Schiff, Grocott-Gomori's methenamine silver, and acid-fast bacilli stains should be performed to rule out microbial infection, such as deep fungal infection, tuberculosis, and leprosy. In addition, examination of the specimen under polarized light microscopy should also be performed as to reveal any foreign body material. These histologic findings are indistinguishable from those of Crohn's disease and may closely resemble sarcoidosis. However, clinical correlation helps in differentiating these conditions.[19,30]

Sarcoidosis

Sarcoidosis is a multiorgan disorder of unknown etiology which usually presents with pulmonary infiltration and hilar lymphadenopathy. Involvement of the eyes, skin, and salivary glands is relatively common. Sarcoidosis rarely involves the oral cavity, although it has been reported to affect the buccal mucosa, tongue, lips, palate, floor of the mouth, mandible, and maxilla. Only 70 well-documented cases of oral sarcoidosis (with jaw bones and salivary glands involvement excluded) had been reported by 2013.[18] Oral manifestations, even though they are rare, could be the first clinical sign of the disease.[31] The gingiva was affected in only four cases.[18] Gingival involvement in sarcoidosis may have many clinical presentations including painless enlargement with or without occasional ulceration, identical to orofacial granulomatosis, or solitary gingival swelling[31] or as gingivitis/periodontitis with bleeding gums.[32] Diagnostic clues in favor of sarcoidosis include the radiographic evidence of lung involvement, increased eosinophil count, and elevated serum ACE levels. In addition, histologic evidence consists of noncaseating granulomatous lesions, accompanied by epithelioid histiocytes rimmed with lymphocytes and scattered Langhans or foreign body-type giant cells. Many cases resolve spontaneously, but if treatment is necessary, it consists mainly of steroids and immune-modulating medications.[32,33]

Crohn's Disease

Crohn's disease is a chronic granulomatous disorder of unknown etiology that affects mainly the ileum but may affect any part of the gastrointestinal tract, including the mouth. The pathogenesis of Crohn's disease is related to the mucosal response to an environmental trigger that can be a bacterium or virus when a genetic predisposition is also present.[34] Oral manifestations are the second most common extraintestinal manifestations of the disease and may precede, occur concurrently, or follow the onset of abdominal symptoms.[35] Oral manifestations include multiple intraoral ulcerations similar to those of aphthous stomatitis, a cobblestone appearance of the buccal mucosa, diffuse firm enlargement of the lips, and reddish granulomatous enlargement of the gingiva. The most frequently affected areas are the lips, buccal mucosa, and gingiva.[36] Orofacial manifestations are identical with those of orofacial granulomatosis, but they are usually associated with active intestinal disease. However, oral lesions precede the abdominal symptoms by months or years in almost 60%, especially in adolescents and young adults.[37] Clinical diagnosis may be challenging if the lesions are subtle in early stages, or in the presence of predominantly gingival involvement. Gingivitis associated with Crohn's disease may appear as gingival erythema or nodular swellings and ulcerations of the gingiva.[34] Clinical differential diagnosis includes other causes of granulomatous gingivitis (foreign body gingivitis, sarcoidosis, and orofacial granulomatosis) and localized juvenile spongiotic gingival hyperplasia (LJSGH) in addition to PCG. Biopsy is necessary to establish diagnosis. Histopathologically, squamous epithelium may present with mild inflammatory cell exocytosis. The connective tissue is fibrous and shows infiltration of lymphocytes and plasma cells. Well-formed granulomas composed of epithelioid histiocytes, and lymphocytes are also seen. The granulomas in orofacial granulomatosis and oral Crohn's disease are similar and the differential diagnosis between the two entities is quite difficult. Therefore, it is important to conduct a thorough clinical investigation to establish the final diagnosis.[30]

Localized Juvenile Spongiotic Gingival Hyperplasia

LJSGH is a recently described benign condition in children and young adults. It was first described by Darling and colleagues, with the proposed term "juvenile spongiotic gingivitis."[38] The current term "Localized juvenile spongiotic gingival hyperplasia" was proposed by Chang and colleagues.[39] However, recently other terms have been also suggested such as "spongiotic gingivitis with odontogenic metaplasia."[40] LJSGH appears as a solitary or multiple gingival lesion(s), with bright red color, on the attached gingiva, with subtly papillary or granular surface.[41,42] The lesions measure 0.2 to 1 cm, develop more often on the labial maxillary gingiva, and bleed easily.[39,42] The lesion is more common in Caucasians and there is no clear gender predominance.[42] LJSGH most commonly appears in children younger than 18 years, age ranged from 5 to 39 year old. However, it is thought that the disease is more frequent at the first 5 years and at the second decade.[42] Differential diagnosis includes pyogenic granuloma, Wegener granulomatosis, foreign body gingivitis, and hypersensitivity reactions including PCG. The etiopathogenesis is not clear. Many factors have been implicated including sex hormones, viruses, mouth breathing, orthodontic treatment, trauma, and developmental abnormalities but no causal relationship has been definitively established.[39,42] Microscopic and immunohistochemical similarities with the junctional epithelium have been reported. It has been proposed that the LJSGH results from "exteriorization" of the junctional epithelium that acquires features associated to the surface epithelium under the influence of local environmental stimuli.[42] Histologically, there is subtle papillary epithelial hyperplasia, spongiosis, interconnecting rete pegs, and inflammatory cell exocytosis. The connective tissue is edematous, with vascular spaces and diffuse inflammatory infiltration.[41] There is no

amelioration with conservative oral hygiene measures or with topical steroids. The best treatment for solitary cases is excision with scalpel or laser. Recent studies showed that cryotherapy could also be efficient for multiple lesions. Recurrence occurs in 5.8% to 28.6% of solitary lesions and in 38.5% of multiple lesions. In some cases, spontaneous remission has been described, probably due to the elimination of a possible unknown causative factor.[42]

Ligneous Gingivitis

Ligneous gingivitis is part of a clinical spectrum of an autosomal recessive condition, characterized by deficiency in plasminogen.[43] Normally when plasminogen is converted to plasmin, it dissolves blood clots. On the deficiency of plasmin formation, blood clots tend to persist and grow and fibrin deposits form plaques and nodules that affect mucosal surfaces. The gingival lesions can present as patchy ulcerated papules and nodules with a very irregular surface. Conjunctival lesions of the upper eye lid that present as creamy yellowish to erythematous lesions are more common. Trauma to mucosal surfaces should be avoided to minimize fibrin accumulation. Topical or systemic plasminogen, or topical heparin combined with prednisone are used to treat the oral lesions. Surgical excision was also reported. The condition is indolent, with no increase in intravascular thrombosis and no effect on life expectancy.[8]

HISTOLOGIC DIFFERENTIAL DIAGNOSIS

Histologic differential diagnosis of PCG can include nonspecific chronic inflammatory conditions, such as chronic periodontitis that is characterized by connective tissue heavily infiltrated with plasma cells, as well as plasma cell neoplasms.[44]

Plasmacytoma

Extramedullary plasmacytoma is a plasma cell neoplasm that develops in tissues other than bone. It is a relatively rare lesion, and it arises in 80% of the cases in nasopharynx, paranasal sinuses, and tonsils.[45] The disease may affect the gingiva but is not that common. Gingival involvement was first described by Martinelli and Rulli[46] as sessile gingival lesion which needs differential diagnosis from chronic gingivitis or PCG.[47] The disease may appear as soft tissue mass that can be asymptomatic or demonstrates spontaneous bleeding. Histologically, the connective tissue is infiltrated by plasma cells in the form of sheets, small islands, or nodules. The plasma cells may vary in size and may be binucleated and multinucleated.[47] These histologic features might not be enough to separate this lesion from PCG. However, the presence of Dutcher bodies and especially the identification of monoclonal Ig expression of these plasma cells are helpful in differential diagnosis. Immunohistochemistry is needed to confirm the monoclonality of the light chains that are expressed in plasmacytomas.[47]

Multiple Myeloma

MM is a systematic disease and is included in malignant monoclonal gammopathies.[48] It is a chronic, malignancy of plasma cells that presents mainly in the bone marrow, but it can also appear in other organs. The clones of plasma cells produce immunologically inactive monoclonal immunoglobulins or their subunits.[49] MM represents 1% of all malignancies and 10% of hematological malignancies.[50,51] The disease develops mostly in patients over 50 year old, with a mean age of 60, and men, especially black men are more commonly involved. The etiopathogenesis of the neoplasm remains unknown. Clinical presentation is the result of the clonal production of plasma cells, the replacement of the normal cells in the bone marrow, and the presence of paraproteins in the urine. Clinical manifestations include bone pain, pathologic fractures, fatigue, amyloidosis, recurrent infections, bleeding predisposition, and nonspecific skin lesions. Diagnostic criteria of MM include the radiographic findings of mild bone resorption, multiple "punched out" radiolucent lesions, or osteoporotic lesions,[52] the presence of atypical plasma cells discovered by bone marrow biopsy and abnormal Immunoglobulins in blood and urine.[53] Oral manifestations develop in around 14% of the patients and include swelling (more often of the mandible), amyloidosis, "punched out" radiolucent lesions in the jaws, tooth mobility, bleeding, and ulcers of the oral mucosa.[53,54] Histologically, there is diffuse infiltration of plasma cells that can vary in appearance and are atypical. Immunohistochemistry is necessary to demonstrate the monoclonal plasma cell nature for the final diagnosis.[53,55]

Leukemic Gingival Infiltration

Both the acute and chronic forms of all types of leukemia may have oral manifestations, but these features are more frequently seen in the acute phase. The oral complications of leukemia are due to the infiltration of leukemic cells that can manifest as gingival enlargement. The enlarged tissues are usually soft, shiny, erythematous, highly tender, and boggy in consistency that can bleed on palpation. The underlying thrombocytopenia can present as petechiae, ecchymosis, and hemorrhage. Neutropenia or impaired granulocyte function can present with increased predisposition to infection and mucosal ulceration.[56,57] Gingival involvement may be the initial presenting symptom in 5% of cases of acute myeloid leukemia.[56] Dreizen and colleagues reported the highest gingival involvement in patients with acute monocytic leukemia (66.7%), followed by acute myelomonocytic leukemia (18.5%), and acute myeloblastic leukemia (3.7%).[58] However, leukemic infiltration is not usually observed in edentulous mucosa. Poor oral hygiene and calculus accumulation may exacerbate the gingival inflammation and bleeding, complicating oral hygiene practice.[59] The diagnosis of leukemia is made by a complete blood count showing pancytopenia and by identifying blast cells in the peripheral blood and bone marrow,[44] whereas the identification of leukemic infiltration in biopsies of oral lesions may lead to diagnosis in undiscovered cases.

Lymphoma

The lymphomas are a group of malignant solid tumors involving cells of the lymphoreticular system. The most common presentation is painless, persistent enlargement of the lymph nodes, but extranodal lesions may also occur, especially in cases of non-Hodgkin lymphoma.[48] Oral lesions as the initial manifestation of the disease are very rare, accounting for 0.1% to 5%.[60] Oral non-Hodgkin lymphoma often mimics inflammatory disease and may present as non-tender gingival swelling with a smooth or ulcerated surface, a mass in the tongue or other oral mucosal sites or as an intraosseous lesion. Oral lesions may be the first manifestation of the disease, but the gingiva is one of the rarest sites for isolated cases (as oppose to palatal mucosa).[60] Radiographic, hematologic, and histopathologic evaluation is required to establish the diagnosis.[44]

SUMMARY

PCG is a benign inflammatory lesion of the gingiva and less often also involving the oral mucosa. Diagnosis is confirmed on clinicopathologic correlation with identification of a dense polyclonal submucosal plasma cell infiltrate. Identifying and preventing exposure to the causative allergen should be always attempted, although it is not always possible as many cases are idiopathic. For chronic symptomatic cases, treatment is directed toward treating symptoms and can range from topical to systemic steroids.

CLINICS CARE POINTS

For diagnosis of plasma cell gingivitis, the following can be noticed:

- Sudden onset of erythematous and edematous lesions of the free and attached gingiva.
- Easily bleeds with a loss of gingival stippling, with or without ulceration.
- Lesions are symptomatic or painful or even burning.

There should be:

- No vesicles, bullae, or Nikolsky sign or Wickham striae of lichenoid lesions.
- No speckled red and white lesions.

CONFLICT OF INTEREST

The authors have no conflict of interest to disclose.

REFERENCES

1. Leuci S, Coppola N, Adamo N, et al. Clinico-Pathological Profile and Outcomes of 45 Cases of Plasma Cell Gingivitis. J Clin Med 2021;10(4). https://doi.org/10.3390/jcm10040830.
2. Kerr DA, McClatchey KD, Regezi JA. Idiopathic gingivostomatitis. Cheilitis, glossitis, gingivitis syndrome; atypical gingivostomatitis, plasma-cell gingivitis, plasmacytosis of gingiva. Oral Surg Oral Med Oral Pathol 1971;32(3):402–23.
3. Solomon LW, Wein RO, Rosenwald I, et al. Plasma cell mucositis of the oral cavity: report of a case and review of the literature. Oral Surg Oral Med Oral Pathol Oral Radiol Endod 2008;106(6):853–60.
4. Mahler V, Hornstein OP, Kiesewetter F. Plasma cell gingivitis: treatment with 2% fusidic acid. J Am Acad Dermatol 1996;34(1):145–6.
5. Román CC, Yuste CM, González MA, et al. Plasma cell gingivitis. Cutis 2002;69(1):41–5.
6. Ferreiro JA, Egorshin EV, Olsen KD, et al. Mucous membrane plasmacytosis of the upper aerodigestive tract. A clinicopathologic study. Am J Surg Pathol 1994;18(10):1048–53.
7. Anil S. Plasma cell gingivitis among herbal toothpaste users: a report of three cases. J Contemp Dent Pract 2007;8(4):60–6.
8. Brad W. Neville CMA, Douglas D. Damm, Angela, et al. Oral Maxillofacial Pathol, 2016: 5-146
9. Smith ME, Crighton AJ, Chisholm DM, et al. Plasma cell mucositis: a review and case report. J Oral Pathol Med 1999;28(4):183–6.
10. Macleod RI, Ellis JE. Plasma cell gingivitis related to the use of herbal toothpaste. Br Dent J 1989;166(10):375–6.
11. Helmy HA, Fadel AF, Mansour KM, et al. Unusual presentation of maxillary plasma cell gingivitis mistakenly treated as aggressive periodontitis. (A case report). Int J Surg Case Rep 2022;93:106998.
12. Chapple ILC, Mealey BL, Van Dyke TE, et al. Periodontal health and gingival diseases and conditions on an intact and a reduced periodontium: Consensus report of workgroup 1 of the 2017 World Workshop on the Classification of Periodontal and Peri-Implant Diseases and Conditions. J Periodontol 2018;89(Suppl 1):S74–84.
13. Jadwat Y, Meyerov R, Lemmer J, et al. Plasma cell gingivitis: does it exist? Report of a case and review of the literature. Sadj 2008;63(7):394–5.
14. Tailor A, Pemberton MN, Murphy R, et al. Plasma cell mucositis related to qat chewing: a report of 2 cases and review of the literature. Oral Surg Oral Med Oral Pathol Oral Radiol 2021;131(3):e65–70.
15. Endo H, Rees TD. Clinical features of cinnamon-induced contact stomatitis. Compend Contin Educ Dent 2006;27(7):403–9 [quiz: 10].
16. Kerr DA, McClatchey KD, Regezi JA. Allergic gingivostomatitis (due to gum chewing). J Periodontol 1971;42(11):709–12.
17. Ranganathan AT, Chandran CR, Prabhakar P, et al. Plasma cell gingivitis: treatment with chlorpheniramine maleate. Int J Periodontics Restorative Dent 2015;35(3):411–3.
18. Kadiwala SA, Dixit MB. Gingival enlargement unveiling sarcoidosis: Report of a rare case. Contemp Clin Dent 2013;4(4):551–5.
19. Lourenço SV, Lobo AZ, Boggio P, et al. Gingival manifestations of orofacial granulomatosis. Arch Dermatol 2008;144(12):1627–30.
20. Kalantzis A, Marshman Z, Falconer DT, et al. Oral effects of low-dose methotrexate treatment. Oral Surg Oral Med Oral Pathol Oral Radiol Endod 2005;100(1):52–62.
21. Yousefi H, Abdollahi M. An Update on Drug-induced Oral Reactions. J Pharm Pharm Sci 2018;21(1):171–83.
22. Vigarios E, Epstein JB, Sibaud V. Oral mucosal changes induced by anticancer targeted therapies and immune checkpoint inhibitors. Support Care Cancer 2017;25(5):1713–39.
23. Moffitt ML, Bencivenni D, Cohen RE. Drug-induced gingival enlargement: an overview. Compend Contin Educ Dent 2013;34(5):330–6.
24. Trackman PC, Kantarci A. Molecular and clinical aspects of drug-induced gingival overgrowth. J Dent Res 2015;94(4):540–6.
25. Le ST, Hinds B, Jordan R, et al. Foreign body gingivitis: An uncommon iatrogenic simulant of oral

lichenoid mucositis. JAAD Case Rep 2019;5(2): 173–5.

26. Gravitis K, Daley TD, Lochhead MA. Management of patients with foreign body gingivitis: report of 2 cases with histologic findings. J Can Dent Assoc 2005;71(2):105–9.

27. Gordon SC, Daley TD. Foreign body gingivitis: clinical and microscopic features of 61 cases. Oral Surg Oral Med Oral Pathol Oral Radiol Endod 1997;83(5):562–70.

28. Ferreira L, Peng HH, Cox DP, et al. Investigation of foreign materials in gingival lesions: a clinicopathologic, energy-dispersive microanalysis of the lesions and in vitro confirmation of pro-inflammatory effects of the foreign materials. Oral Surg Oral Med Oral Pathol Oral Radiol 2019;128(3):250–67.

29. Bansal M, Singh N, Patne S, et al. Orofacial granulomatosis affecting lip and gingiva in a 15-year-old patient: A rare case report. Contemp Clin Dent 2015; 6(Suppl 1):S94–6.

30. Müller S. Non-infectious Granulomatous Lesions of the Orofacial Region. Head Neck Pathol 2019; 13(3):449–56.

31. Tripathi P, Aggarwal J, Chopra D, et al. Sarcoidosis presenting as isolated gingival enlargement: a rare case entity. J Clin Diagn Res 2014;8(11):Zd25–6.

32. Bouaziz A, Le Scanff J, Chapelon-Abric C, et al. Oral involvement in sarcoidosis: report of 12 cases. Qjm 2012;105(8):755–67.

33. Agrawal AA. Gingival enlargements: Differential diagnosis and review of literature. World J Clin Cases 2015;3(9):779–88.

34. Woo VL. Oral Manifestations of Crohn's Disease: A Case Report and Review of the Literature. Case Rep Dent 2015;2015:830472.

35. Skrzat A, Olczak-Kowalczyk D, Turska-Szybka A. Crohn's disease should be considered in children with inflammatory oral lesions. Acta Paediatr 2017; 106(2):199–203.

36. Laube R, Liu K, Schifter M, et al. Oral and upper gastrointestinal Crohn's disease. J Gastroenterol Hepatol 2018;33(2):355–64.

37. Plauth M, Jenss H, Meyle J. Oral manifestations of Crohn's disease. An analysis of 79 cases. J Clin Gastroenterol 1991;13(1):29–37.

38. Darling MR, Daley TD, Wilson A, et al. Juvenile spongiotic gingivitis. J Periodontol 2007;78(7): 1235–40.

39. Chang JY, Kessler HP, Wright JM. Localized juvenile spongiotic gingival hyperplasia. Oral Surg Oral Med Oral Pathol Oral Radiol Endod 2008; 106(3):411–8.

40. Theofilou VI, Pettas E, Georgaki M, et al. Localized juvenile spongiotic gingival hyperplasia: Microscopic variations and proposed change to nomenclature. Oral Surg Oral Med Oral Pathol Oral Radiol 2021;131(3):329–38.

41. Solomon LW, Trahan WR, Snow JE. Localized juvenile spongiotic gingival hyperplasia: a report of 3 cases. Pediatr Dent 2013;35(4):360–3.

42. Siamantas I, Kalogirou EM, Tosios KI, et al. Spongiotic Gingival Hyperplasia Synchronously Involving Multiple Sites: Case Report and Review of the Literature. Head Neck Pathol 2018;12(4):517–21.

43. MacPherson M, Pho M, Cox J, et al. Ligneous gingivitis secondary to plasminogen deficiency: a multidisciplinary diagnostic challenge. Oral Surg Oral Med Oral Pathol Oral Radiol 2020;130(3):e87–95.

44. Harris NL, Jaffe ES, Diebold J, et al. The World Health Organization classification of hematological malignancies report of the Clinical Advisory Committee Meeting, Airlie House, Virginia, 1997. Mod Pathol 2000;13(2):193–207.

45. Trivedi S, Dixit J, Goel MM. Extramedullary plasmacytoma of the gingiva. BMJ Case Rep 2016;2016. https://doi.org/10.1136/bcr-2015-211606.

46. Martinelli C, Rulli MA. Primary plasmacytoma of soft tissue (gingiva). Report of a case. Oral Surg Oral Med Oral Pathol 1968;25(4):607–9. published Online First: Epub Date]|.

47. Webb CJ, Makura ZG, Jackson SR, et al. Primary extramedullary plasmacytoma of the tongue base. Case report and review of the literature. ORL J Otorhinolaryngol Relat Spec 2002;64(4):278–80 [published Online First: Epub Date]|.

48. Abdelwahed Hussein MR. Non-Hodgkin's lymphoma of the oral cavity and maxillofacial region: a pathologist viewpoint. Expert Rev Hematol 2018; 11(9):737–48 [published Online First: Epub Date]|.

49. Ozaki M, Yamanaka H. A case of IgD myeloma with extraosseous spread to the gingiva. Oral Surg Oral Med Oral Pathol 1988;65(6):726–30 [published Online First: Epub Date]|.

50. Currie WJ, Hill RR, Keshani DK. An unusual cause of maxillary tuberosity enlargement. Br Dent J 1994; 177(2):60–2.

51. Kyle RA, Gertz MA, Witzig TE, et al. Review of 1027 patients with newly diagnosed multiple myeloma. Mayo Clin Proc 2003;78(1):21–33.

52. Mozaffari E, Mupparapu M, Otis L. Undiagnosed multiple myeloma causing extensive dental bleeding: report of a case and review. Oral Surg Oral Med Oral Pathol Oral Radiol Endod 2002; 94(4):448–53.

53. Rajkumar SV, Dimopoulos MA, Palumbo A, et al. International Myeloma Working Group updated criteria for the diagnosis of multiple myeloma. Lancet Oncol 2014;15(12):e538–40.

54. Epstein JB, Voss NJ, Stevenson-Moore P. Maxillofacial manifestations of multiple myeloma. An unusual case and review of the literature. Oral Surg Oral Med Oral Pathol 1984;57(3):267–71.

55. Lee SH, Huang JJ, Pan WL, et al. Gingival mass as the primary manifestation of multiple myeloma:

report of two cases. Oral Surg Oral Med Oral Pathol Oral Radiol Endod 1996;82(1):75–9.

56. Hasan S, Khan NI, Reddy LB. Leukemic gingival enlargement: Report of a rare case with review of literature. Int J Appl Basic Med Res 2015;5(1):65–7.

57. Tefferi A, Pardanani A. Myeloproliferative Neoplasms: A Contemporary Review. JAMA Oncol 2015;1(1):97–105.

58. Dreizen S, McCredie KB, Keating MJ, et al. Malignant gingival and skin "infiltrates" in adult leukemia. Oral Surg Oral Med Oral Pathol 1983;55(6):572–9.

59. Lim HC, Kim CS. Oral signs of acute leukemia for early detection. J Periodontal Implant Sci 2014; 44(6):293–9.

60. Manjunatha BS, Gowramma R, Nagarajappa D, et al. Extranodal non-Hodgkin's lymphoma presenting as gingival mass. J Indian Soc Periodontol 2011;15(4):418–20.

Fungal Lesions of the Oral Mucosa Diagnosis and Management

Tina R. Woods, DMD[a],*, Jamie White, DMD[b], Ioannis Koutlas, DDS, MS[c]

KEYWORDS

- Oral fungal infection • Candidiasis • Histoplasmosis • Mucormycosis • Blastomycosis
- Coccidioidomycosis • Cryptococcosis • Aspergillosis

KEY POINTS

- Candidiasis is a superficial and most common fungal infection.
- Most deep fungal infections are uncommon.
- Immunosuppressed individuals with deep fungal infections experience more severe, often life-threatening disease, and early diagnosis and appropriate treatment are imperative.

CANDIDIASIS

Pathogenesis

Candidiasis is caused by the *Candida* species, a dimorphic group of fungi that can exist both in yeast and mold form.[1] *Candida* species are found in soil, food, and the human body, and are accepted as members of the normal oral flora in an estimated 30% to 60% of healthy individuals.[2,3] *Candida albicans* is the most common species found in the oral cavity.

Disease-causing candidal overgrowth can be encountered with the use of broad-spectrum antibiotics and corticosteroids (including inhaled steroids), in denture wearers with poor oral hygiene, xerostomic patients, and immunocompromised individuals with human immunodeficiency virus (HIV), uncontrolled diabetes, individuals undergoing chemo- and/or radiotherapy and transplant patients.[3] Children with undeveloped immune systems may be susceptible to candida overgrowth.[3–6] Candidiasis may be localized or disseminated, depending on the state of the host's immune system and mucosal barriers.[2]

Clinical Features

Pseudomembranous candidiasis ("thrush") is the most common form featuring white wipeable patches often revealing an erythematous mucosa (**Fig. 1**).[5–7] It commonly affects the dorsal tongue, buccal mucosa, palate, and oropharynx.[6–8] The other forms of candidiasis mostly show erythematous lesions and include acute atrophic candidiasis, median rhomboid glossitis, chronic multifocal candidiasis, angular cheilitis, and denture stomatitis (chronic atrophic candidiasis).[6] In acute atrophic candidiasis, the oral mucosa appears red and the tongue shows atrophic areas with loss of filiform papillae (**Fig. 2**), necessitating the differentiation from other possible causes of atrophic glossitis such as vitamin/nutrient deficiencies.[6,7] Patients often present with a burning sensation of the oral mucosa.

Median rhomboid glossitis appears as an erythematous patch on the midline of the posterior tongue dorsum characterized by loss of the filiform papillae (**Fig. 3**).[9,10] This presentation is often asymptomatic and observed in individuals who

[a] Oral and Maxillofacial Pathology, Department of Stomatology, James B. Edwards College of Dental Medicine, 173 Ashley Avenue, Suite 344, MSC 507, Charleston, SC 29425, USA; [b] Oral and Maxillofacial Pathology, Department of Oral Maxillofacial Surgery and Pathology, University of Mississippi Medical Center, School of Dentistry, 2500 North State Street, Jackson, MS 39216, USA; [c] Division of Oral and Maxillofacial Pathology, University of Minnesota School of Dentistry, Malcom Moos Health Sciences Tower, 515 Delaware Street, Southeast, Minneapolis, MN 55455, USA
* Corresponding author.
E-mail address: woodsti@musc.edu

Oral Maxillofacial Surg Clin N Am 35 (2023) 271–281
https://doi.org/10.1016/j.coms.2022.10.004
1042-3699/23/© 2022 Elsevier Inc. All rights reserved.

smoke and/or use steroid inhalers.[10] It may influence the development of another clinical presentation termed *chronic multifocal candidiasis* if contact with the palate leads to palatal involvement.[6]

Angular cheilitis may occur as part of chronic multifocal candidiasis or alone, presenting as erythematous lesions with commissural fissuring and crusting (**Fig. 4**).[6,7] Causes include reduced vertical dimension resulting in accentuated skin folds allowing collection of saliva in the area, thus providing a moist environment for *Candida* to thrive.[5] Individuals who habitually lick their lips and bite the corners of their mouths can also develop such lesions.[10] Angular cheilitis may be caused solely by *C albicans* or in combination with *Staphylococcus aureus* or by *S aureus* alone.[6,10] As in acute atrophic candidiasis, it is pertinent to exclude other factors for the development of these lesions such as vitamin and nutritional deficiencies.[5,6]

Use of dentures for prolonged periods of time combined with poor oral hygiene or ill-fitting prostheses may create an environment fostering candidal overgrowth. This is termed denture stomatitis, or *chronic atrophic candidiasis*, and presents as erythematous mucosa in the area covered by a removable prosthesis.[3,8]

A less common presentation that is white, does *not* wipe off, and is often more localized is chronic hyperplastic candidiasis (candidal leukoplakia), usually occurring on the anterior buccal mucosa and lateral border of tongue.[7,9] According to some investigators, such lesions may represent leukoplakias suprainfected with candida organisms. Candida can induce epithelial hyperplasia and hyperkeratosis. Lesions of hyperplastic candidiasis can also present as speckled white and red areas (speckled leukoplakia). Chronic hyperplastic candidiasis may be associated with an increased risk for the development of oral dysplastic lesions and candida is often seen accompanying dysplastic and cancerous oral lesions.[9]

Lastly, *chronic mucocutaneous candidiasis* is a rare form in which individuals develop persistent candida infections of not only the oral mucosa but other mucous membranes, skin, hair, and nails as part of a distinct immunologic disorder. Some patients may also have endocrine abnormalities, iron-deficiency anemia or autoimmune polyendocrinopathy, candidiasis, and ectodermal dystrophy (APECED) syndrome.[2]

Diagnosis

The classic clinical presentation of candidiasis is often diagnostic but can be confirmed by exfoliative cytology, culture, or mucosal biopsy.[11] Culturing is considered the most sensitive method.[12] However, culturing of clinical lesions unrelated to *Candida* can still identify the presence of *Candida* as this organism is often part of normal oral flora.[3] Cytologic smears are beneficial, cost-effective, noninvasive diagnostic tools in certain clinical settings, especially in erythematous candidiasis. Microscopically, *Candida* organisms show 2 to 6 μm hyphae and yeasts (pseudohyphae), with special stains Grocott–Gomori methenamine silver (GMS) and periodic acid-Schiff (PAS) used to highlight yeast spores and hyphae.[2,12] Lesions of chronic hyperplastic candidiasis are expected to resolve *after* antifungal therapy.[3]

Management

Use of clotrimazole troches (10 mg, 5x daily for 7–14 days) or cream, or nystatin rinse (4–6 mL 4x daily for 7–14 days) can address mild candidiasis.[13] Patients with angular cheilitis may benefit from the application of clotrimazole cream.[6] Moderate to severe candidiasis can be treated with oral fluconazole (100–200 mg daily for 7–14 days).[13] Itraconazole solution (200 mg once daily for up to 28 days) is used for candidiasis nonresponsive to fluconazole.[13]

Rinsing with water or saline after the use of corticosteroid inhalers should decrease the incidence of candidal infection.[2,5] In addition to oral antifungal therapy, patients with candida-associated denture stomatitis should adopt improved hygiene practices of thoroughly disinfecting their dentures twice a day and removing them while sleeping.[5,13] Of benefit will be applying antifungal cream to the intaglio surface of the denture (1% Clotrimazole OTC cream, 2–4 x daily).[3] Fabrication of new dentures may be necessary if prostheses are ill-fitting and above recommendations do not lead to improvement.

HISTOPLASMOSIS
Pathogenesis

Histoplasmosis is an endemic fungal infection caused by *Histoplasma capsulatum*, a dimorphic fungus native to and localized within the geographic regions of the Ohio and Mississippi River valleys in the United States, as well as in Mexico and Central and South America.[14,15] *Histoplasma capsulatum* is naturally found in moist, warm, and nitrogen-rich soil, such as in areas containing bird or bat-disturbed soil. Inhalation of spores initiates lung infection.[14,15] After transforming from conidia, yeast cells are phagocytized in their primary host cell (the macrophage) where they reside and remain localized to the lungs or

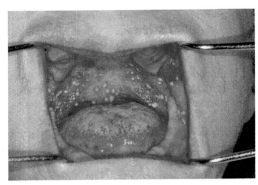

Fig. 1. Pseudomembranous candidiasis. (*Courtesy of* Donald M. Cohen, DMD, MS, MBA; Indraneel Bhattacharyya, DDS, MSD; and Nadim M. Islam, DDS, BDS, Gainesville, FL.)

disseminate.[15] Residing in macrophages is considered an important ability of *H capsulatum* to survive and spread throughout the body.[16]

Clinical Features

When infection occurs, both the patient's immune status and intensity of exposure to the fungal organisms determine symptoms and severity of the illness.[15,17] An exposed individual may be asymptomatic if exposure to the fungal organisms is low; however, if high, symptoms will likely develop. Patients may present with a self-limited form of acute pulmonary histoplasmosis characterized by flu-like symptoms such as fever, headache, myalgia, cough, and chest pain.[15] Lung involvement presenting as calcified hilar lymph nodes or pulmonary infiltrates may be observed radiographically.[6] Immunocompromised individuals who have acquired the organisms may develop reactivation of infection and expression of disease as pulmonary or extrapulmonary.[16] A less common manifestation of disease seen in such patients is chronic histoplasmosis and closely resembles tuberculosis.[18]

Dissemination of disease may occur during the first few weeks after acute infection.[17] Oral lesions of histoplasmosis reportedly occur in 20% to 76% of patients with progressive disseminated histoplasmosis, although they may occur in all forms of infection.[14,18] These lesions present as indurated ulcers with rolled borders, similar in appearance to squamous cell carcinoma, or as nodules and granulomatous lesions of the tongue, palate, gingiva, and buccal mucosa (**Figs. 5–7**).[14,19]

Diagnosis

Diagnostic tools include microscopic examination, culture, and serology. When possible, histopathologic examination of tissue is recommended. Special stains GMS and PAS readily disclose *H capsulatum* characterized by small 2 to 4 μm, oval, narrow-based budding yeasts.[15] Blood culture using the lysis-centrifugation method has improved sensitivity and can rapidly detect *H capsulatum* in disseminated disease or enzyme immunoassay (EIA) to detect *Histoplasma* antigen in serum and urine.[14,15,20]

Management

Acute histoplasmosis is self-limiting with most cases resolving without therapy. For progressive disseminated histoplasmosis of mild-to-moderate severity, itraconazole (200 mg 3x/day) for 3 days and then twice daily for at least 12 months is recommended.[17] For moderately severe to severe disseminated disease, liposomal Amphotericin B (3.0 mg/kg daily) is recommended for 1 to 2 weeks, followed by oral itraconazole (200 mg 3x/day) for 3 days and then 200 mg twice daily for a total of at least 12 months. For immunosuppressed patients who cannot be reversed or relapsed cases, lifelong therapy with itraconazole (200 mg daily) may be required. The level of itraconazole in the blood should be evaluated to ensure adequate drug exposure.[17]

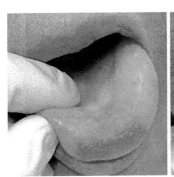
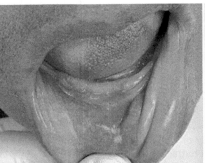
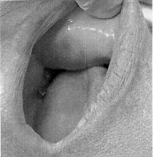

Fig. 2. Atrophic candidiasis. (*Courtesy of* Daniel Mandic, DDS, Jackson, MS; *with permission.*)

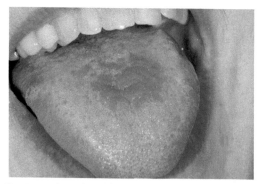

Fig. 3. Median rhomboid glossitis. (*Courtesy of* Donald M. Cohen, DMD, MS, MBA; Indraneel Bhattacharyya, DDS, MSD; and Nadim M. Islam, DDS, BDS, Gainesville, FL; *with permission.*)

MUCORMYCOSIS (ZYGOMYCOSIS)

Mucormycosis represents a group of mycoses causing morbidity and mortality due to relentless progressive invasion of affected tissues especially if driven by an underlying predisposing condition. The term zygomycosis that includes both mucormycosis and entomophthoramycosis (a tropical infection) has been used interchangeably with the term mucormycosis, especially in individuals with rhinocerebral disease.[21]

Pathogenesis

Humans are constantly exposed to and acquire mucormycosis via direct skin/mucosa penetration or inhalation of fungal spores. Inhalation can lead to sinus, orbital, nasal, central nervous system (CNS) or pulmonary infections. Risk factors for the development of mucormycosis include: (1) diabetic ketoacidosis (causing most often rhinocerebral infection), leading to dissociation of iron from

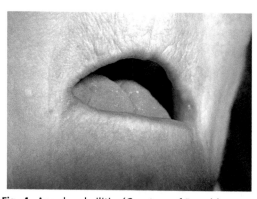

Fig. 4. Angular cheilitis. (*Courtesy of* Donald M. Cohen, DMD, MS, MBA; Indraneel Bhattacharyya, DDS, MSD; and Nadim M. Islam, DDS, BDS, Gainesville, FL; *with permission.*)

sequestering proteins and resulting in enhanced fungal survival and virulence, (2) solid-organ and hematopoietic stem cell transplantation, (3) defects in phagocytic function such as in patients with neutropenia or treated with high-dose glucocorticoids, (4) hemodialysis and chelation therapy leading to increased free iron delivered to the fungus, (5) penetrating trauma/burns and (6) use of intravenous catheters and moist dressings causing macerated skin.[22] Rhino-orbital-cerebral mucormycosis has emerged as a suprainfection in patients with coronavirus disease-2019 (COVID-19), especially in India.[23] It is unclear if the virus predisposes patients to the fungal infection or if the infection is a consequence of another underlying cause in patients with COVID-19, such as diabetes mellitus and use of corticosteroids.

Clinical Features

In the maxillofacial region, mucormycosis presents as a rhino-orbital-cerebral and cutaneous disease. Patients may initially present with nonspecific dull sinus pain, nasal stuffiness/congestion, pain affecting the eyes, blurry vision, and cutaneous cellulitis. Fever may occur in 50% of the patients.[22] Nasal involvement can extend intraorally causing swelling of the maxillary alveolus and palate, leading to tissue ulceration and necrosis, occasionally with black coloration (**Fig. 8**). If patients are not treated or treatment is delayed, extension of disease can involve the ethmoid sinus and the orbits causing proptosis with chemosis, diplopia, and loss of vision. Lesions can also involve the trigeminal/facial/orbital/optic nerves and cavernous sinus.[22] Progression of disease varies, which may be related to the site of infection, species, and the patients' immunocompetence. Although some patients deteriorate in days, it may take months to years for lethal progression if untreated.

Diagnosis

Orofacial and maxillary involvement is best diagnosed by tissue biopsy in concordance with computed tomography (CT) and MRI to better visualize bone involvement and soft tissue extension, respectively.[22] Histopathology with special stains GMS and PAS allow identification of the characteristic 10 to 30 μm thick-walled nonseptate and branching at right angles hyphae.

Management

Antifungal treatment with debridement of necrotic tissue is essential for the management of mucormycosis in conjunction with reversal of underlying predisposing factors. Delaying chemotherapy treatment of underlying malignancy or

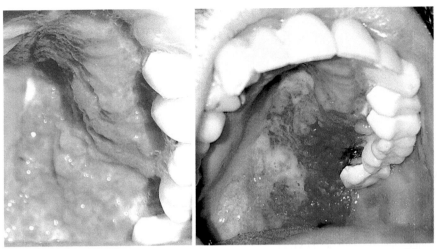

Fig. 5. Histoplasmosis presenting as a granular and ulcerated lesion of the left palate in a middle-aged patient with liver and endocrine comorbidities. (*Courtesy of* Stephen H. Roth, DDS, New York, NY; *with permission*.)

transplantation, before mucormycosis is eradicated, is not advised.[22] Monitoring chemotherapy and immunosuppression during antifungal treatment is recommended.

First-line treatment of mucormycosis is Amphotericin B, 1 to 1.5 mg/kg once per day for Amphotericin B lipid complex or 5 mg/kg once a day for liposomal Amphotericin B, the latter being less toxic and with better CNS penetration.[22] Posaconazole or isavuconazole have been used as alternatives to Amphotericin B as salvage therapy in individuals with refractory disease or as stepdown therapy in those who have shown improvement with Amphotericin B. In one study, an experimental combination of polyenes with echinocandins has shown promising results in murine mucormycosis.[24] However, breakthrough mucormycosis has been described in patients receiving posaconazole, isavuconazole, or echinocandin prophylaxis.[22] Limited data from uncontrolled

studies have provided support for hyperbaric oxygen therapy in combination with antifungal therapy and surgery, due to the fungistatic action of hyperbaric oxygen resulting in enhanced wound healing and neutrophilic action.[22]

ASPERGILLOSIS

Aspergillosis is caused by many species of *Aspergillus* manifesting either as invasive infections or as noninvasive allergies or clusters of fungal organisms (mycetoma)in normal individuals. It is the second most common opportunistic fungal infection after candidiasis. The infective species can grow at 37°C; however, some species can cause allergic respiratory response without this ability.[25] Among the many species, *A fumigatus* is the most common form causing both invasive infections, chronic disease and most allergic responses, whereas *A flavus* causes a higher number of sinus, cutaneous, and eye infections.[25] Asthmatics may experience episodes of attacks and may develop an invasive, potentially destructive infection of nasal and cranial structures. The prevalence has increased in recent years with cases encountered in intensive care units, in individuals with severe influenza, severe COVID-19 who primarily develop lung disease, and in patients with chronic obstructive pulmonary disease.[25,26]

Pathogenesis

Aspergillus species have worldwide distribution and are found in soil, water, air (indoor and outdoor), in bedding, and organic decaying vegetation. The most common modes for conidia to

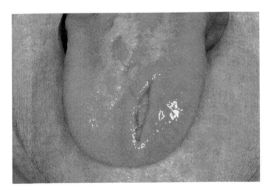

Fig. 6. Histoplasmosis. (*Courtesy of* Donald M. Cohen, DMD, MS, MBA; Indraneel Bhattacharyya, DDS, MSD; and Nadim M. Islam, DDS, BDS, Gainesville, FL.)

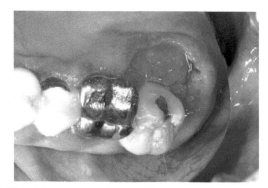

Fig. 7. Histoplasmosis presenting as a nonhealing ulceration in the area of recently extracted tooth #1. (*Courtesy of* Donald M. Cohen, DMD, MS, MBA; Indraneel Bhattacharyya, DDS, MSD; and Nadim M. Islam, DDS, BDS, Gainesville, FL; *with permission.*)

enter is through inhalation or from nail infection (onychomycosis). Most immunocompetent individuals will not develop clinical respiratory disease; however, propensity for disease increases exponentially with higher numbers of conidia, as in moldy or dusty environments (construction or remodeling). Rhinosinusitis is the most common form of infection, and risk for infection increases in immunosuppressed individuals, diabetics, and individuals with improper ciliary function of the respiratory tract.[25] The incubation period for invasive aspergillosis varies from 2 to 90 days, the time needed for the spores to enlarge, germinate and disseminate. Allergic responses may exacerbate with continuous or repeated exposure.

Clinical Features

Aspergillus rhinosinusitis may present with headache, fever, nasal congestion, purulent or bloody nasal discharge, and occasionally facial swelling. Aspergillosis should be suspected in recurrent sinusitis refractory to antibiotic therapy. Oral disease is uncommon, observed primarily in immunosuppressed individuals, and usually affects the gingiva that becomes edematous with a grayviolaceous coloration (**Fig. 9**). When untreated, ulcerations develop followed by necrotic eschars. Dental procedures such as extractions or endodontic treatment, especially in the posterior maxillary dentition potentially introduce the fungus to the maxillary sinus. In immunosuppressed individuals and in diabetics, oral lesions of Aspergillosis often occur as a spectrum of upper or lower respiratory disseminated disease and may present as extension from contiguous structures such as the maxillary sinus to the palate. Vascular invasion progresses to bone and orofacial soft tissue destruction. Saprophytic infection of sinuses may

manifest as a fungus mass (mycetoma and aspergilloma) and may show calcifications.

Diagnosis

Diagnostic methods include histopathologic evaluation of lesional tissue to identify septate 3 to 4 μm hyphae with dichotomus branching at acute angles. However, identification by histomorphology is only suggestive as other fungal organisms have a similar microscopic appearance, Adetection for identification of galactomannan release by Aspergillus organisms or protein antigen, culture, and real-time PCR[25] are more definitive.

Management

Antifungal triazoles (voriconazole, posaconazole) are preferred agents with echinocandins (caspofungin, micafungin) and Amphotericin B second-line agents. Management of patients with invasive disease may require antifungal therapy with aggressive surgical debridement of necrotic tissue. For individuals with allergic fungal sinusitis, corticosteroids with debridement may be necessary. Immunosuppressed individuals with disseminated disease often have contracted aspergillosis in a nosocomial environment and have a poorer prognosis. Prevention from spore inhalation via masks and HEPA filters are recommended for all, especially when exposed to an environment where high numbers of spores is unavoidable.

BLASTOMYCOSIS

Blastomycosis is an endemic systemic fungal infection with most cases in North America caused by the dimorphic fungi *Blastomyces dermatitidis* and *B gilchristii*.[27] The geographic distribution of most cases overlaps with that of histoplasmosis but extends further north.[6] These areas include south, central, southeastern and midwestern United States, Canadian provinces bordering the Great Lakes, and areas along the St. Lawrence River.[15,27,28] It is reported to be endemic to Africa and related to *B percursus* and *B emzantsi*.[15,28]

Pathogenesis

Blastomyces dermatitidis can be found in decaying organic matter such as in soil, leaf litter, and wood.[14,15] Interaction with such soil or recreational activities leads to aerosolized conidia of *B dermatitidis* being inhaled.[15] Once organisms reach the lung, they convert to yeast form which provides an advantage of the organism with its larger size not easily ingested by phagocytes.[16]

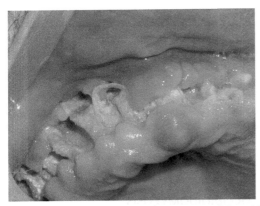

Fig. 8. Maxillary mucormycosis. (*Courtesy of* Donald M. Cohen, DMD, MS, MBA; Indraneel Bhattacharyya, DDS, MSD; and Nadim M. Islam, DDS, BDS, Gainesville, FL.)

Clinical Features

Severity of symptoms depends on the amount of exposure and the patient's immune status.[15] The degree of illness ranges from subclinical infection to varying degrees of pneumonia.[27] Less than half of infected individuals have symptomatic disease.[15] Interestingly, blastomycosis is uncommon among immunocompromised individuals, such as organ transplant recipients and those with AIDS. However, when it occurs in this population, it is more frequently disseminated and has a poorer prognosis.[6,15,27]

Although blastomycosis usually presents as localized pulmonary disease, 25% to 40% of

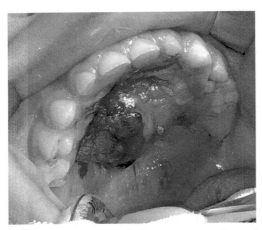

Fig. 9. Aspergillosis manifesting as a 2 cm × 3 cm ulcerated swelling of the palate in a 5-year-old immunocompetent child. (*Reprinted* with permission from Elsevier. The Lancet Infectious Diseases, 2020; 20(2):260.)

patients develop extrapulmonary disseminated disease.[27] Patients with pulmonary blastomycosis are often asymptomatic or present with flu-like illness.[15] Individuals with severe infection may have symptoms resembling pneumonia with high fever, cough and lung infiltrate.[15] With dissemination, two-thirds of individuals show the involvement of skin, bone, genitourinary tract, abdominal organs, CNS, and oropharyngeal mucosa.[6,15,27] Oral manifestations of blastomycosis are rare and may be due to extrapulmonary dissemination or local direct inoculation.[6,19] Oral lesions may present anywhere appearing as ulcerations, granulomatous lesions, verrucous-sessile lesions or as intrabony abscesses.[7,14,20] Ulcerative lesions of blastomycosis may appear irregular with rolled borders mimicking squamous cell carcinoma.[6,19,20]

Diagnosis

Diagnosis is made by microscopic examination that reveals granulomatous inflammation with multinucleated giant cells containing spherical, broad-based budding yeast cells 8 to 15 μm in diameter with a thick double-contoured, refractive wall easily detected on hematoxylin and eosin preparations and auxiliary GMS and PAS special stains.[6,15] Although the growth of these organisms in culture is slow and requires approximately 4 weeks or more, it is the most accurate and sensitive diagnostic method and should be performed for confirmation.[6,15,27] Serologic tests lack sensitivity and specificity.[15,27]

Management

Healthy patients with mild, acute, self-limited pulmonary blastomycosis may not require treatment as infection may resolve spontaneously.[22,27] Immunocompromised patients can develop moderate to severe pneumonia or disseminated disease requiring antifungal therapy.[15,27] Mild-to-moderate pulmonary and disseminated extrapulmonary blastomycosis are treated with oral itraconazole (200 mg, 3x per day) for 3 days and then once or twice per day for 6 to 12 months.[27] For moderately severe to severe pulmonary blastomycosis or moderately severe to severe disseminated extrapulmonary blastomycosis, a lipid formulation of Amphotericin B (3-5 mg/kg per day) for 1 to 2 weeks, or until improvement is noted, followed by oral itraconazole (200 mg, 3x per day) for 3 days, and then 200 mg twice per day, for a total of 6 to 12 months.[27] In all cases, serum levels of itraconazole should be evaluated after 2 weeks to ensure adequate drug exposure.[27]

Immunosuppressed patients may require lifelong suppressive therapy with oral itraconazole.

CRYPTOCOCCOSIS

Cryptococcosis is an invasive global opportunistic fungal infection with two complex species, *Cryptococcus neoformans,* and *C* gattii, which cause human disease from spore inhalation. *C neoformans* accounts for approximately 80% of all cases, causes meningoencephalitis, and has a predilection for immunocompromised patients. *C gatti* compromises 20% of cases, causes pulmonary infections, and has a predilection for immunocompetent individuals.[29]

Pathogenesis

Cryptococcus neoformans is found in avian excreta, soil, and trees (bark, trunk hollows, decaying wood).[30] Once restricted to eucalyptus trees in tropical and subtropical climates, *C gatti* has been identified globally, possibly due to climate changes and ecological shifts.[31]

Cryptococcal spores are surrounded by a mucopolysaccharide capsule aiding in resistance to antifungal medications. Although the primary site infected is the lung, dissemination may include the CNS, viscera, bone, skin, and rarely oral mucosa.[30] Latent infections may occur in association with immunosuppression.[29]

Clinical Features

Cryptococcosis is the most common cause of meningitis associated with HIV/AIDS worldwide, especially in sub-Saharan Africa. Most patients present with headaches (75%), followed by fever, cranial nerve palsy, neck stiffness, seizures, lethargy, memory loss, and coma.[32,33] Pulmonary cryptococcosis may present as acute respiratory distress syndrome (ARDS), cough, dyspnea, chest pain, hemoptysis, and constitutional symptoms. Mucocutaneous lesions may present as nodular-granulomatous masses, pustules, papules, or as superficial or deep ulcerations and cellulitis.[32] Oral cryptococcosis is rare and may represent the first sign of disseminated infection, presenting as ulcers or granulomatous lesions of the tongue, palate, gingiva, and mandible (**Fig. 10**).[34,35]

Diagnosis

Diagnosis is made by tissue biopsy, serology, culture, and radiographic imaging. Histopathological examination reveals small round-ovoid spores 4 to 6 μm in diameter surrounded by a clear capsule that can be visualized with mucicarmine special stain.[6]

Management

Treatment is often multidisciplinary and dependent on the immune status of the patient and clinical presentation (pulmonary only vs disseminated disease with or without CNS involvement). Mild-to-moderate disease without CNS involvement is usually treated with fluconazole for a period of 4 to 6 months and in severe cases with Amphotericin B for 4 to 6 weeks. Immunocompromised patients may require more aggressive treatment with lifelong fluconazole maintenance.[29]

COCCIDIOIDOMYCOSIS

Coccidioidomycosis (valley fever) is an endemic mycosis caused by the dimorphic fungi *Coccidioides immitis* and *C posadasii* found in semiarid climates of the Southwestern United States, Central America, and South America.[36] *C. immitis* is prevalent in California, extending eastward into the states of Arizona and Utah, whereas *C posadasii* is found predominantly in Arizona, New Mexico, Nevada, Texas, Mexico, Central and South America.[37] Most cases in North America are from California and Arizona.

Pathogenesis

The fungi remain stable in dry desert soil for years but soil disruption (earthquakes, dust storms, forest fires, excavation) can release them into the air and can be inhaled.[37]

Clinical Features

Among individuals with infection, 60% are asymptomatic or show self-limiting respiratory symptoms, whereas 40% present with pulmonary and systemic symptoms 1 to 3 weeks post-exposure.[36] Less than 1% may develop disseminated disease, with cutaneous involvement being the most frequent extrapulmonary manifestation, involving the face and the extremities. Tongue and lip ulcerations are observed in approximately 20% of cases (**Fig. 11**).[38] Underlying skeletal and bone involvement may present as osteomyelitis or multiple bone abscesses.[39]

Diagnosis

Diagnosis is based on histopathologic examination of tissue, serology, and fungal cultures. Histopathology reveals large 20 to 60 μm round spherules, many containing endospores, and can be highlighted with GMS and PAS special stains.[6] A coccidioides EIA of serum has a rapid turnaround time and 90% sensitivity in moderate to severe cases.[37]

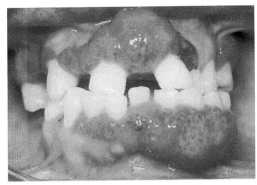

Fig. 10. Cryptococcal infection showing ulcerated granulomatous maxillary and mandibular gingiva. (*From* Delgado WA, Romero de Leon E. 14th International Congress IAOP/AAOMP Clinical Pathology Conference Case 6. *Head Neck Pathol.* 2008;2(4):298-301.)

Management

Self-limiting cases involve regular follow-up care to monitor symptoms. For moderate infections, azoles remain the first line of therapy, usually fluconazole (400 mg/d) or itraconazole (400 mg/d) for 3 to 6 months or longer. Amphotericin B is reserved for more severe or refractory cases.[40]

PARACOCCIDIOIDOMYCOSIS

Paracoccidioidomycosis (formerly also known as South American blastomycosis) is the most common invasive mycosis endemic to subtropical humid areas of Latin America and caused by dimorphic soil-inhabiting fungus *Paracoccidioides brasiliensis* with a 50% to 75% prevalence of infected individuals in those areas.[41,42]

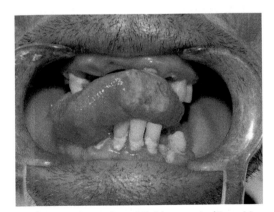

Fig. 11. Disseminated coccidioidomycosis. (*From* Mendez LA, Flores SA, Martinez R, de Almeida OP. Ulcerated Lesion of the Tongue as Manifestation of Systemic Coccidioidomycosis. *Case Rep Med.* 2017;2017:1489501.)

Pathogenesis

Affected individuals often are involved in agriculture. The disease is self-limiting in most immunocompetent individuals. Most cases initially present as upper or lower respiratory disease which can spread via lymphatics or hematogenously to lymph nodes.

Clinical Features

Most primary infections are subclinical. There are two clinical forms, acute/subacute and chronic, and an asymptomatic form. Children and adolescents usually present with the acute/subacute form, representing 10% of all clinical cases. Most patients are middle-aged and, the vast majority are males (15:1). In females, it is believed there is inhibition of mycelial-to-yeast conversion by estrogens.[43] As with other fungal infections, severity is variable. Transplant patients, individuals taking immunosuppressant medications, and patients with HIV/AIDS may experience severe disseminated disease or reactivation of infection.

Oral lesions can be multifocal, fungating, indurated or ulcerated and affect both masticatory and nonmasticatory mucosa. Ulcerations may occur also around the mouth and nose, in the pharynx and larynx. Individuals with lung involvement may present with patchy pneumonia.

Diagnosis

Diagnosis is obtained serologically with immunodiffusion assays,[44] which are inexpensive and have a high specificity (95%) and sensitivity (80%). Tissue biopsy reveals round, thick-walled yeast cells 15 to 30 μm in diameter and up to 60 μm in some cases with multiple budding yeasts present within multinucleated giant cells as a component of granulomatous inflammation.[42] Special stains GMS and PAS readily disclose the characteristic yeast and buds. Fungal culture is not recommended due to slow growth of the fungus.

Management

Patients with mild-to-moderate disease are treated with itraconazole 200 to 400 mg daily for up to a year. With more advanced disease, Amphotericin B followed by itraconazole may be required. Oral voriconazole (6 mg/kg/d for 6 to 12 months) has been successfully used in cases with CNS involvement.[42] Patients on antifungal prophylaxis with itraconazole or voriconazole have an increased risk for the development of mucormycosis.

SUMMARY

Clinical presentations of oral fungal infections are variable and may mimic other pathology, including diseases presenting with multiple ulcerations or even malignancies. A thorough medical history followed by prompt biopsy of suspicious (especially multiple or indurated) ulcers and following proper surgical and radiographic protocols will aid in early detection, diagnosis and increased survival rates for patients.

CLINICS CARE POINTS

- Many fungal organisms have a similar microscopic appearance therefore diagnosis of serious fungal infections must be confirmed by culture and/or specific tests.
- Candida can induce epithelial hyperplasia and hyperkeratosis and is often seen accompanying dysplastic and cancerous oral lesions
- Rhino-orbital-cerebral mucormycosis has emerged as a suprainfection in patients with coronavirus disease-2019.
- Aspergillosis is the second most common opportunistic fungal infection and should be suspected in recurrent sinusitis refractory to antibiotic therapy
- Deep fungal infections often clinically resemble malignancies

DISCLOSURE

The authors have no conflict of interest.

REFERENCES

1. Murray P, Rosenthal K, Pfaller M. Fungal classification, structure, and replication. In: Murray P, Rosenthal K, Pfaller M, editors. Medical microbiology. 9th edition. Philadelphia: Elsevier; 2021. p. 572–7.
2. Kosmidis C, Denning DW. Opportunistic and systemic fungi. In: Cohen J, Powderly WG, Opal SM, editors. Infectious diseases. 4th edition. China: Elsevier; 2017. p. 1681–709.
3. Hellstein JW, Marek CL. Candidiasis: red and white manifestations in the oral cavity. Head Neck Pathol 2019;13(1). https://doi.org/10.1007/s12105-019-01004-6.
4. Murray PR, Rosenthal KS, Pfaller MA. Opportunistic mycoses. In: Murray PR, Rosenthal KS, Pfaller MA, editors. Medical microbiology. 9th edition. Philadelphia: Elsevier; 2021. p. 649–74.
5. Simon L, Silk H. Diseases of the mouth. In: Kellerman RD, Rakel DP, editors. Conn's current therapy 2022. Philadelphia: Elsevier; 2022. p. 1048–53.
6. Neville B, Damm D, Allen C, et al. Fungal and protozoal diseases. In: Neville B, Damm D, Allen C, et al, editors. Oral and maxillofacial pathology. 4th edition. Canada: Elsevier; 2016. p. 191–9.
7. Bandara HMHN, Samaranayake LP. Viral, bacterial, and fungal infections of the oral mucosa: Types, incidence, predisposing factors, diagnostic algorithms, and management. Periodontol 2000 2019;80(1):148–76.
8. Lombardi A, Ouanounou A. Fungal infections in dentistry: Clinical presentations, diagnosis, and treatment alternatives. Oral Surg Oral Med Oral Pathol Oral Radiol 2020;130(5):533–46.
9. Vila T, Sultan AS, Montelongo-Jauregui D, et al. Oral candidiasis: a disease of opportunity. J Fungi (Basel) 2020;6(1):15.
10. Millsop JW, Fazel N. Oral candidiasis. Clin Dermatol 2016;34(4):487–94.
11. Rajendra Santosh AB, Muddana K, Bakki SR. Fungal infections of oral cavity: diagnosis, management, and association with COVID-19. SN Compr Clin Med 2021;3(6):1373–84.
12. Murray P, Rosenthal K, Michael P. Laboratory diagnosis of fungal disease. In: Murray P, Rosenthal K, Pfaller M, editors. Medical microbiology. 9th edition. Philadelphia: Elsevier; 2021. p. 589–99.
13. Pappas PG, Kauffman CA, Andes DR, et al. Clinical practice guideline for the management of candidiasis: 2016 update by the infectious diseases society of America. Clin Infect Dis 2015;62(4):e1–50.
14. Telles DR, Karki N, Marshall MW. Oral fungal infections: diagnosis and management. Dent Clin North Am 2017;61(2):319–49.
15. Murray P, Rosenthal K, Pfaller M. Systemic mycoses caused by dimorphic fungi. In: Murray P, Rosenthal K, Pfaller M, editors. Medical microbiology. 9th edition. Philadelphia: Elsevier; 2021. p. 632–48.
16. Murray P, Rosenthal K, Pfaller M. Pathogenesis of fungal disease. In: Murray P, Rosenthal K, Pfaller M, editors. Medical microbiology. 9th edition. Philadelphia: Elsevier; 2021. p. 578–86.
17. Wheat LJ, Freifeld AG, Kleiman MB, et al. Clinical practice guidelines for the management of patients with histoplasmosis: 2007 update by the Infectious Diseases Society of America. Clin Infect Dis 2007;45(7):807–25.
18. Mutalik VS, Bissonnette C, Kalmar JR, et al. Unique oral presentations of deep fungal infections: a report of four cases. Head Neck Pathol 2021;15(2):682–90.
19. Fitzpatrick SG, Cohen DM, Clark AN. Ulcerated lesions of the oral mucosa: clinical and histologic review. Head Neck Pathol 2019;13(1):91–102.
20. Thompson GR, Le T, Chindamporn A, et al. Global guideline for the diagnosis and management of the

endemic mycoses: an initiative of the European Confederation of Medical Mycology in cooperation with the international society for human and animal mycology. Lancet Infect Dis 2021;21(12):e364–74.

21. Davies GE, Thornton CR. Development of a monoclonal antibody and a serodiagnostic lateral-flow device specific to *Rhizopus arrhizus* (Syn. *R. oryzae*), the principal global agent of mucormycosis in humans. J Fungi (Basel) 2022;8(7):756.

22. Spellberg B, Ibrahim AS. Mucormycosis. In: Loscalzo J, Fauci A, Kasper D, et al, editors. Harrison's principles of internal medicine 21e. McGraw Hill; 2022. Available at: https://accesspharmacy.mhmedical.com/content.aspx?bookid=3095&sectionid=265435350. Accessed August 01, 2022.

23. Pal R, Singh B, Bhadada SK, et al. COVID-19-associated mucormycosis: an updated systematic review of literature. Mycoses 2021;64(12):1452–9.

24. Ibrahim AS, Gebremariam T, Fu Y, et al. Combination echinocandin-polyene treatment of murine mucormycosis. Antimicrob Agents Chemother 2008;52(4):1556–8.

25. Denning DW. Aspergillosis. In: Loscalzo J, Fauci A, Kasper D, et al, editors. Harrison's principles of internal medicine 21e. McGraw Hill; 2022. Available at: https://accesspharmacy.mhmedical.com/content.aspx?bookid=3095&sectionid=265435278. Accessed August 01, 2022.

26. Shishido AA, Mathew M, Baddley JW. Overview of COVID-19-associated invasive fungal infection. Curr Fungal Infect Rep 2022;1–11. https://doi.org/10.1007/s12281-022-00434-0. PMID 35846240.

27. Chapman SW, Dismukes WE, Proia LA, et al. Clinical practice guidelines for the management of blastomycosis: 2008 update by the Infectious Diseases Society of America. Clin Infect Dis 2008;46(12):1801–12.

28. Cornely OA, Alastruey-Izquierdo A, Arenz D, et al. Global guideline for the diagnosis and management of mucormycosis: an initiative of the European Confederation of Medical Mycology in cooperation with the Mycoses Study Group Education and Research Consortium. Lancet Infect Dis 2019;19(12):e405–21.

29. Casadevall A. Cryptococcosis. In: Loscalzo J, Fauci A, Kasper D, et al, editors. Harrison's principles of internal medicine 21e. McGraw Hill; 2022. Available at: https://accesspharmacy.mhmedical.com/content.aspx?bookid=3095&sectionid=265435208. Accessed August 01, 2022.

30. Kwon-Chung KJ, Fraser JA, Doerlng TL, et al. Cryptococcus neoformans and Cryptococcus gattii, the etiologic agents of cryptococcosis. Cold Spring Harb Perspect Med 2014;4(7):a019760.

31. Gushiken AC, Saharia KK, Baddley JW. Cryptococcosis. Infect Dis Clin North Am 2021;35(2):493–514.

32. Nemade SV, Shinde KJ. Cryptococcosis. In: Granulomatous diseases in otorhinolaryngology, head and neck. Singapore: Springer; 2021. https://doi.org/10.1007/978-981-16-4047-6_17.

33. Rajasingham R, Smith RM, Park BJ, et al. Global burden of disease of HIV-associated cryptococcal meningitis: an updated analysis. Lancet Infect Dis 2017;17(8):873–81.

34. Delgado W. Oral Cryptococcosis. JSM Trop Med Res 2017;2(1):1015.

35. DiNardo AR, Schmidt D, Mitchell A, et al. First description of oral cryptococcus neoformans causing osteomyelitis of the mandible, manubrium and third rib with associated soft tissue abscesses in an immunocompetent host. Clin Microbiol Case Rep 2015;1(3):017. PMID: 27227123; PMCID: PMC4876986.

36. Laniado-Laborin R, Alcantar-Schramm JM, Cazares-Adame R. Coccidioidomycosis: an update. Curr Fungal Infect Rep 2012;6:113–20.

37. Bajwa AK, Rongkavilit C. Update on coccidioidomycosis in the United States and beyond. Glob Pediatr Health 2020;7. https://doi.org/10.1177/2333794X20969282. 2333794X20969282.

38. Filho D, Deus AC, Meneses Ade O, et al. Skin and mucous membrane manifestations of coccidioidomycosis: a study of thirty cases in the Brazilian states of Piauì and Maranhão. An Bras Dermatol 2010;85(1):54–61.

39. Reed D, Kostosky N, Epstein A, et al. Disseminated coccidioidomycosis with orbital osteomyelitis and periorbital abscess. Ophthal Plast Reconstr Surg 2021;37(5):e173–6.

40. Limper AH, Knox KS, Sarosi GA, et al. An official American thoracic society statement: treatment of fungal infections in adult pulmonary and critical care patients. Am J Respir Crit Care Med 2011;183(1):96–128.

41. Travassos LR, Taborda CP, Colombo AL. Treatment options for paracoccidioidomycosis and new strategies investigated. Expert Rev Anti Infect Ther 2008;6(2):251–62.

42. Thompson GR 3rd, Le T, Chindamporn A, et al. Global guideline for the diagnosis and management of the endemic mycoses: an initiative of the European Confederation of Medical Mycology in cooperation with the International Society for Human and Animal Mycology. Lancet Infect Dis 2021;21(12):e364–74 [published correction appears in Lancet Infect Dis. 2021 Nov;21(11):e341].

43. Blotta MH, Mamoni RL, Oliveira SJ, et al. Endemic regions of paracoccidioidomycosis in Brazil: a clinical and epidemiologic study of 584 cases in the southeast region. Am J Trop Med Hyg 1999 Sep;61(3):390–4.

44. Perenha-Viana MC, Gonzales IA, Brockelt SR, et al. Serological diagnosis of paracoccidioidomycosis through a Western blot technique. Clin Vaccin Immunol 2012;19(4):616–9.

Moving?

Make sure your subscription moves with you!

To notify us of your new address, find your **Clinics Account Number** (located on your mailing label above your name), and contact customer service at:

Email: journalscustomerservice-usa@elsevier.com

800-654-2452 (subscribers in the U.S. & Canada)
314-447-8871 (subscribers outside of the U.S. & Canada)

Fax number: 314-447-8029

Elsevier Health Sciences Division
Subscription Customer Service
3251 Riverport Lane
Maryland Heights, MO 63043

*To ensure uninterrupted delivery of your subscription, please notify us at least 4 weeks in advance of move.